the JCAHO Mock Survey

Made Simple

1999 Edition

Kathryn A. Chamberlain, CPHQ

Candace J. Hamner, RN, MA

Opus Communications
Marblehead, MA

The JCAHO Mock Survey Made Simple, 1999 Edition is published by Opus Communications.

Copyright 1999 by Opus Communications, Inc.
Cover image © 1999 PhotoDisc, Inc.

In some cases, the assessment points in this book have been summarized from the JCAHO's *Comprehensive Accreditation Manual for Hospitals (CAMH)*. Be sure to refer to the standards and scoring guidelines in the CAMH for a full description of JCAHO requirements and other examples of compliance with the standards.

All rights reserved. Printed in the United States of America.   5 4 3 2 1

ISBN 1-57839-050-8

No part of this publication may be reproduced, in any form or by any means, without prior written consent of Opus Communications or the Copyright Clearance Center (978/750-8400). Please notify us immediately if you have received an unauthorized copy.

Opus Communications provides information resources for the health care industry. A complete listing of our newsletters and books is found at the back of this book.

Opus Communications is not affiliated in any way with the Joint Commission on Accreditation of Healthcare Organizations.

Jennifer I. Cofer, Executive Publisher
Rob Stuart, Vice President/Publisher
Kristen Woods, Executive Editor
Brooke Husbands, Associate Editor
Candace J. Hamner, RN, MA, Co-Author
Kathryn A Chamberlain, CPHQ, Co-Author
Jean St. Pierre, Art Director
Mike Mirabello, Graphic Designer
Shane Katz, Cover Designer

Advice given is general. Readers should consult professional counsel for specific legal, ethical, or clinical questions.

Arrangements can be made for quantity discounts. For more information contact:
Opus Communications
P.O. Box 1168
Marblehead, MA 01945
Telephone: 800/650-6787 or 781/639-1872
Fax: 781/639-2982
E-mail: customer_service@opuscomm.com

Visit the Opus Communications web site: www.opuscomm.com

Table of Contents

About the Authors iv
Preface v
Introduction: Managing your mock survey and evaluating your results vii

Mock Survey Basics
  Pre-Survey Checklist: Accreditation Participation Requirements 1
  Checklist 1: Patient Rights and Organization Ethics (RI) 7
  Checklist 2: Patient Assessment (PE) 17
  Checklist 3: Care of the Patient (TX) 25
  Checklist 4: Patient and Family Education (PF) 35
  Checklist 5: Continuum of Care (CC) 39
  Checklist 6: Performance Improvement (PI) 45
  Checklist 7: Leadership (LD) 53
  Checklist 8: Environment of Care (EC) 61
  Checklist 9: Human Resources (HR) 69
  Checklist 10: Information Management (IM) 75
  Checklist 11: Infection Control (IC) 89
  Checklist 12: Governance (GO) 95
  Checklist 13: Management (MA) 99
  Checklist 14: Medical Staff (MS) 103
  Checklist 15: Nursing (NR) 117

Common Trouble Spots
  Checklist 16: Staff Competency 121
  Checklist 17: Credentialing 127
  Checklist 18: Medical Records 133
  Checklist 19: Physicians' Offices and Ambulatory Care Sites 153
  Checklist 20: IV Conscious Sedation vs. Anesthesia 169
  Checklist 21: Restraint and Seclusion 173
  Checklist 22: Equipment and Utility Preventative Maintenance 187
  Checklist 23: The Seven Environment of Care Plans 193

Self-Assessments
  Checklist 24: CEO's Responsibilities 207
  Checklist 25: Department Managers' Responsibilities 213
  Checklist 26: Medical Staff Leaders' Responsibilities 225
  Checklist 27: Line Staff's Responsibilities 233

About the Authors

Kathryn A. Chamberlain, CPHQ, has more than 25 years of health care management experience with the North Shore Medical Center in Salem, Massachusetts, a Partners (Massachusetts General Hospital/Brigham and Women's Hospital) affiliate. For the past seven years, she managed the organization's performance improvement, utilization management, and accreditation activities, which culminated in accreditation with commendation. She was also instrumental in the start-up of the North Shore Health System, an integrated health care organization, and was responsible for developing its Medical Management Program. She is currently self-employed as a health care consultant.

Candace J. Hamner, RN, MA, has been actively involved in JCAHO survey preparation since 1981 in four different hospitals. Currently, she is the Vice President of Care Management for Northwest Hospital Center, a LifeBridge Health center, in Randallstown, Maryland. In this role, she serves as the hospital's safety officer and JCAHO survey coordinator, and oversees the hospital's quality and performance improvement, JCAHO accreditation, utilization review, risk and claims management, medical records, patient satisfaction, social work, and medical staff office activities. Northwest Hospital Center achieved accreditation with commendation in its last two JCAHO surveys.

Preface

If your hospital is one of the over 15,000 health care organizations in the United States that are striving to achieve accreditation from the Joint Commission on Accreditation of Healthcare Organizations (JCAHO), you understand that survey preparation can be not only a chore but also an overwhelming challenge. Somehow, in addition to all of your other responsibilities, you need to verify that all of your hospital's policies, procedures, medical records, and other documents are in line with the JCAHO's standards and practiced as written, and that each person in the hospital, from the line staff to your CEO, can confidently answer any JCAHO-related questions surveyors might pose during their rounds.

Whether your upcoming JCAHO survey will be your first or one of many in a long history of surveys, your goal is the same—to achieve accreditation with commendation. And the best way to ensure that you've met all of the JCAHO's requirements is to conduct a mock survey ideally 12 months before your surveyors' visit. Your mock survey is by far the most important survey preparation activity you will undertake. This thorough assessment of your current level of JCAHO compliance will help you to pinpoint which areas of your hospital are in line with JCAHO requirements, and which fall short of the mark. This way you can effectively channel your hospital's resources and energies into correcting known problems areas, instead of wasting a lot of time concentrating on issues that don't need additional attention.

We designed *The JCAHO Mock Survey Made Simple* to help you effectively conduct such a mock survey. We waded through the JCAHO's *Comprehensive Accreditation Manual for Hospitals (CAMH)* and created easy-to-understand assessment points for you to use to gauge your hospital's level of compliance with the standards. The workbook contains three sections:

- *Mock Survey Basics*—includes checklists focusing on each of the chapters in the *CAMH*;
- *Common Trouble Spots*—concentrates on common Type I issues, such as restraint and seclusion, IV conscious sedation, and equipment and utility preventative maintenance; and
- *Self Assessments*—offers tools each key player in your JCAHO survey can use to test their familiarity with JCAHO requirements.

In each of these checklists, you'll find succinct examples of compliance for each assessment point, drawn directly from our own experiences as JCAHO survey coordinators. As you read through these examples, keep in mind that they are only *examples* of compliance, and are not in any way JCAHO requirements. There are a number of ways to demonstrate compliance with each standard, and there is no one "right answer." Each hospital could conceivably have a different example of compliance, and all of these examples could very well meet surveyors' approval.

Perhaps most importantly, we've added a "Fast Track" feature for hospitals who may not have the time to conduct a full-blown mock survey and gauge their compliance with each assessment point

Preface

in this workbook. We understand that every hospital has a different schedule and set of priorities, and we've left it up to you to decide just how intensive you want your mock survey to be. If you're pressed for time, first gauge your compliance with all of the assessment points marked with a "fast track" icon 🏃. These are the issues which surveyors will most likely give the most scrutiny. Then, if once you've completed this initial high-priority assessment, you find that you have some additional time, go back and assess your compliance with the issues you skipped over during your first pass. This way your improvement teams can start correcting major problems before they address minor compliance issues.

We hope that you find *The JCAHO Mock Survey Made Simple* a useful tool and that you use it to make your upcoming JCAHO survey the best one you've had yet!

Kathryn A. Chamberlain, CPHQ
Health Care Consultant
Gloucester, Massachusetts

Candace J. Hamner, RN, MA
Vice President, Care Management
Northwest Hospital Center
Randallstown, Maryland

Introduction: Managing your mock survey and evaluating your results

As more hospitals recognize the importance of achieving the Joint Commission on Accreditation of Healthcare Organizations' (JCAHO) award of accreditation with commendation, their survey coordinators' roles are becoming increasingly vital. But that doesn't mean that the job is getting any easier! Somehow, survey coordinators need to find the time to ensure that all of their hospitals' documents, systems, and personnel are compliant with JCAHO requirements—a daunting task to say the least.

Most survey coordinators confront this challenge by conducting mock surveys. During these "practice runs," managers and other key staff members play the roles of surveyors and assess the entire hospital's compliance with the JCAHO's standards. This mock survey should be as thorough as possible. Your surveyors should look for evidence that all of the JCAHO's requirements have been met, and ensure that staff throughout the organization can confidently discuss how they work to keep the hospital in compliance. Evidence of compliance can be found in hospital documentation, staff interviews, and even discussions with patients and their families. Anything that will help prove to the Joint Commission that you have a quality organization should be identified.

In this section, we've outlined the basic steps you need to follow as you manage your mock survey. Use these guidelines as you walk through the mock survey process, but don't feel that you have to blindly follow them. Remember that you know your organization and its culture best, and only you can decide how to meet the needs of your hospital.

Step 1: Develop your mock survey approach and schedule

In an ideal world, your hospital would have only two priorities—providing perfect patient care and achieving accreditation with commendation. But in reality, most health care organizations always have a number of major initiatives in the works at once, and you need to find a way to squeeze your JCAHO mock survey into the hospital's overtaxed agenda.

About a year before your scheduled survey, make a list of all of the major issues that the hospital is scheduled to tackle in the coming year. Estimate just how much time the hospital realistically will have to devote to its mock survey and whether you should hold a "comprehensive" or a "fast track" mock survey.

A comprehensive mock survey uses all of the checklists in this book and will take approximately three months to complete, from training your mock surveyors to analyzing their findings. Then, depending on what types of compliance problems you uncover, it might take a month or longer to correct all of the identified problems. While such a survey is a major time commitment for any organization, particularly when the hospital has other strategic issues competing for its time, it is definitely worth the effort. It focuses your entire organization on JCAHO compliance, and will help to teach staff JCAHO requirements.

Introduction: Managing your mock survey and evaluating your results

If after you review your hospital's upcoming agenda you discover that you only have a minimum of time to devote to your mock survey, you should consider holding a "fast track" survey. In this type of a survey, you'll have your mock survey teams sweep through all of the common JCAHO trouble spots. We've highlighted all of these trouble spots with a "fast track" icon on the checklists 🏃. This will help you to ensure that you're in compliance with all of the JCAHO's key requirements. Once you're done with this cursory review, you can always go back later and focus on additional assessment points. As a general rule, a fast track survey would be appropriate for an organization which

- is short on time (e.g., it has less than one year until its survey),
- is focused on numerous other priorities, or
- has a strong year-round survey preparation program.

But, a fast track mock survey is not as thorough as a comprehensive mock survey and won't help you to heighten JCAHO-awareness throughout the hospital, since it involves just a few members of the organization.

Whichever survey approach you choose, it is important to develop a schedule to communicate your expectations to the rest of the organization. Determine when you'll conduct your mock survey, when the results need to be compiled and summarized, and how long you have to spend correcting compliance problems. See the sample timeline in Figure 1 for a suggested schedule.

Step 2: Form mock survey teams

Once you've decided whether you'll hold a comprehensive or a fast track mock survey and developed a corresponding time line, your next step is to decide how many mock survey teams you will need, and who should be on each one.

You should assign a mock survey team to handle each checklist in this book, but this doesn't necessarily mean that you'll need to form 27 individual teams. Consider assigning several related checklists to a single survey team. For example, a team with information management expertise could easily assess the organization's compliance with the hospital's IM standards and review all of your medical records. Or, a patient care team might take on both the patient assessment (PE) and care of the patient (TX) standards. In some instances, you may have "teams" already in place in the form of committees. For example, an information steering committee may be perfect for assessing compliance with the information management (IM) standards.

However you decide to break down the work load, your mock surveyors' responsibilities will be the same—they'll canvass the organization and assess each department's compliance with their assigned standards, as applicable. For instance, the mock survey team responsible for assessing compliance with the JCAHO's patient rights and organization ethics (RI) standards will gauge every department's compliance and consistency with those JCAHO's standards.

Ideal mock survey team members are typically managers and key staff who have knowledge and expertise in the areas covered by the standards and who have been through a JCAHO survey. No matter what type of expertise these survey team members have, they should all be detail oriented, good communicators, and committed to a successful JCAHO survey. And a good sense of humor won't hurt either!

Figure 1

Comprehensive Mock Survey Timeline

SURVEY

Task	\multicolumn{12}{c	}{Time to survey in months}
	12	11	10	9	8	7	6	5	4	3	2	1
Determine mock survey approach	✓											
Select mock surveyors	✓											
Train mock surveyors	✓											
Conduct mock survey and monitor progress		✓										
Collect and analyze findings			✓									
Communicate findings to leaders			✓									
Assign improvement projects			✓									
Perform improvement projects			✓	✓	✓	✓	✓	✓	✓	✓	✓	✓
Track results of improvement projects				✓	✓	✓	✓	✓	✓	✓	✓	✓
Communicate progress to staff and leaders				✓	✓	✓	✓	✓	✓	✓	✓	✓
Evaluate success of improvement projects										✓		
Follow-up on any remaining problems											✓	✓

Introduction: Managing your mock survey and evaluating your results

Be sure to speak with your potential survey team members' supervisors to explain the mock survey process and what a team member's responsibilities will be *before* you assign anyone any work. These managers may need to give their staff members time away from their other duties to participate in the mock survey, and therefore you'll need their full support.

It's always wise to assign a leader to each survey team to keep the group focused and on track, too. Try to select leaders who have experience managing people and who have influence in your organization. This type of person will have the interpersonal skills and organizational pull you'll need to make sure the job gets done. See Figure 2 for a list of suggested mock survey team leaders.

And don't forget to set completion times for the teams! You don't want your assessments to drag on, since you really should devote most of your time to correcting compliance problems.

Step 3: Train the mock survey teams

The hospital will invest a lot of time, effort, and resources in your mock survey, and therefore you want to ensure that the survey team members understand exactly what it is they are supposed to do. Be sure to give them a little more direction than simply ripping out the checklists in this book, handing them out, and telling them to "go for it!" You need quality results, and any time spent up front explaining the mock survey process and answering team members' questions will be well invested.

First, explain to the team members how to look at the hospital as an outsider, and not with their "employee" eyes. For example, they should get into the habit of asking themselves questions like

- What do the corridors really look like? Are they cluttered with equipment and furniture?
- How would a local resident find out about our community lecture series?
- How easy is it for a physician to find the information he or she needs in the medical record?
- What would it be like to be a non-English speaking patient in our hospital?
- How good are our directions to Radiology?
- What have we done in the last 18 months that we're really proud of and that customers would see as significant performance improvements?

If each team member thinks this way and digs for information, they'll gather valuable data during their assessments which you can later use to set your improvement priorities and develop corrective action plans.

Next, you should teach the team members how to use the checklists in this book. If you're having a "fast track" survey, explain that they should only gauge compliance with the highlighted assessment points 🏃. If you have the time for a comprehensive survey, instruct them to judge the hospital's compliance with each and every assessment point on the checklists. It might be worth the effort to review a few assessment points with them, too, to teach them what constitutes compliance in the JCAHO's eyes, and what doesn't. Review the basic mock survey tactics listed in Figure 3 with them as well.

Finally, remind the team members that the examples of compliance on each checklist are not JCAHO requirements, but are merely examples designed to help them better understand what can demonstrate compliance to the JCAHO. And, you should explain that many times one item can demonstrate compliance with a number of JCAHO standards. For example, your hospital's weekly

Figure 2

Suggested Mock Survey Team Leaders

Assessment Team	Suggested Leader(s)
Patient Rights and Organization Ethics (RI)	VP of patient services, COO, or ethics committee chair
Patient Assessment (PE)	A well-organized director of a nursing or patient care department
Care of the Patient (TX)	VP of patient services, medical director, chief or director of surgery, or the chief or director of anesthesia
Patient and Family Education (PF)	A well-organized nurse or clinician, knowledgeable in patient education. Supported by an interested MD.
Continuum of Care (CC)	VP or director of nursing or director of case management
Performance Improvement (PI)	Director of PI or the chair of the quality council
Leadership (LD)	COO, CEO, or survey coordinator
Environment of Care (EC)	VP of operations or safety committee chair
Human Resources (HR)	VP or director of human resources
Information Management (IM)	Director of medical records or computer services, VP responsible for information services, or a member of the medical staff or nursing
Infection Control (IC)	Director or chair of infection control committee
Governance (GO)	CEO or survey coordinator
Management (MA)	CEO, COO, or survey coordinator
Medical Staff (MS)	President of the medical staff
Nursing (NR)	Nurse executive or survey coordinator
Staff Competency	HR director, staff education director, or anyone responsible for assessing and documenting staff competency
Credentialing	Medical staff coordinator, chair of the medical staff committee, president of the medical staff, or the medical director
Medical Records	A member of the medical records committee or the group that performs quarterly medical records reviews

Figure 2 (cont'd)

Suggested Mock Survey Team Leaders (cont'd)	
Assessment Team	**Suggested Leader(s)**
Physicians' Offices/Ambulatory Care Sites	Practice manager, director of ambulatory department, or medical director of ambulatory department
IV Conscious Sedation vs. Anesthesia	Manager or medical director of any location where conscious sedation or anesthesia is administered
Restraint and Seclusion	Nurse managers or medical directors of any locations where restraint is used
Equipment and Utility Preventative Maintenance	Manager of facilities or biomedical engineering or safety officer
The Seven Environment of Care Plans	Survey coordinator, safety officer, VPs responsible for environment of care, biomedical engineering, plant operations, facilities engineering, infection control, and environmental services

bulletin may offer readers safety tips, explain the hospital's mission and vision, and offer news about upcoming service expansions or community education classes, and therefore demonstrate compliance with some of the JCAHO's environment of care and leadership standards.

Step 4: Conduct the mock survey and monitor the teams' progress

Once you've organized and trained your survey teams, it's time to put them to work. Make sure that each team is familiar with its responsibilities and time frame for completion, and then send them all out into your hospital to conduct their assessments. These assessments should take about a month to complete.

But this doesn't mean your job is finished. As the teams make their way through the hospital analyzing all of your documentation and systems for compliance with the JCAHO's standards, they'll still need your support and guidance. Touch base with the mock survey team leaders at least once a week to find out how the work is progressing and to offer advice if needed. Regardless of how you follow-up with the teams, whether it's in weekly meetings, during phone conversations, or via e-mail updates, it is important that you keep the lines of communication open. Don't wait until the last minute to find out that a few teams are lagging behind or have gotten off track. This will put your schedule in jeopardy.

Each time you speak to your team leaders, look for answers to questions such as

- What problems are the teams encountering?
- What can I do to help?
- Are the departments cooperating with the survey teams?
- Are the teams maintaining our set schedule?

Figure 3

Basic Mock Survey Tactics

Remind your mock survey teams to look for the following items as they gauge the hospital's compliance with the standards. If they keep these reference points in mind as they conduct their assessments, they'll gather the information you need to determine what the hospital's compliance problems are, and how you should correct them.

Consistency
The JCAHO requires you to provide patients with one consistent level of care throughout your organization. Be sure to look closely at all of the hospital's policies and procedures and make sure that they are followed consistently in all departments. For example, your policy and procedure for conscious sedation must be applied consistently at all locations where conscious sedation is administered, such as in endoscopy, radiology, and patient care units.

Integration
Joint Commission surveyors want to see that your hospital uses tools and processes that encourage departments to work together. For example, your medical records should be patient-focused and not discipline focused. Therefore, an endoscopy record might include a patient's nursing assessment, anesthesia assessment, physician procedure notes, and recovery and discharge instructions all on one form. Medical records that consist of multiple pieces of paper, each telling only one chapter of a patient's care, won't demonstrate integration of care to surveyors.

Collaboration
Collaboration means that each person in the hospital draws from the knowledge of his or her co-workers to offer patients better quality care, such as when nutrition and nursing staff work together to develop an assessment tool to help caregivers screen for nutritionally at-risk patients. As the survey teams assess the hospital, they should ensure that there are no barriers, or at least minimal barriers, between all departments, divisions, medical staff services, senior management, and staff.

By keeping your finger on the pulse of the survey, you can quickly identify and eliminate all problems.

Step 5: Collect and analyze the teams' results

After all of the survey teams have completed their assessments, you and your survey team leaders will need to sit down and read through all of the teams' results and identify your hospital's compliance problems.

About one week before the survey teams' results are due, schedule a meeting with your survey team leaders to teach them how to analyze their results. You might want to offer them an analysis tool, such as the one in Figure 4 to help them organize their data and highlight all of the hospital's weak points. Explain to the leaders that they should flip through each of their assigned checklists and identify each assessment point which received a "no" and was therefore identified as non-compliant.

Introduction: Managing your mock survey and evaluating your results

Figure 4

Mock Survey Results Analysis Tool

Directions: Use this form to help you organize the results of your mock survey assessments, determine which problems are priorities, and brainstorm on potential solutions. Complete one of these forms for each of the checklists you completed during your mock survey. Rate the priority of each problem using the following scale: A=urgent/E=low priority.

Checklist Title: _____

Standard(s) not met	Issue(s)	Department(s) Involved	Priority Level (circle one)	Suggested Actions
			A B C D E	
			A B C D E	
			A B C D E	
			A B C D E	
			A B C D E	
			A B C D E	

As they record these problem areas on your analysis tool (Figure 4), ask the team leaders to note which problems they feel are of particular concern. They might want to use the "fast track" icons on the checklists as a general indicator of which areas are extremely important and deserve immediate attention, but they might also have their own thoughts on which areas are key improvement priorities for your organization.

This analysis should take the team leaders about a month to complete. After they're finished, collect all of the completed checklists and the team leaders' analyses. Place the completed checklists in a binder for future reference, and begin to read through the team leaders' suggested improvement priorities.

As you read through the team leaders' suggested improvement priorities, rank them according to level of urgency. We suggest you use the following guidelines to help you determine which problems need immediate attention, and which are lesser priorities:

- Level of compliance—Are you completely non-compliant with a JCAHO requirement, or do you just need to do a little work to bring the hospital into compliance?
- Importance of the problem—Has the issue been a past surveyor "hot button?" Was it identified as a problem during your last survey?
- How long it will take to correct—Will it take two to three months or two to three weeks to correct?

Once you've developed your list of the top problems, discuss it with the hospital's leadership. Bring them up-to-date on the organization's level of survey readiness, and explain just how much work you think it will take to get the hospital in compliance before the real JCAHO surveyors arrive. Together, you should develop a definitive list of improvement priorities.

Step 6: Implement corrective action plans

From your list of approved improvement priorities, you should break down the improvement projects into two categories: Those that can be easily resolved by a department manager and those that will require a team effort.

Hand off any improvement projects that can be easily resolved by a department manager, and explain to this individual what needs to be done, when it needs to be completed, and offer some advice on how it can best be accomplished. Keep a log (see Figure 5) of what projects you have delegated to department managers, and note the deadline for each project. You can use this list to help you and your executive management team keep track of the status of all of your corrective action plans.

Next, organize improvement teams to address multidisciplinary compliance problems, such as developing a hospital-wide policy on restraint and seclusion, developing a hospital-wide patient and family education program, or establishing a staff competency program. The key here is to identify issues which are hospital-wide, affect multiple departments, and will need input and cooperation from several different areas to solve the problem.

Use our improvement project log (see Figure 5) to note which departments are involved in each problem, and select individuals from these departments to join your improvement mock teams, or assign these tasks to your mock survey teams. You may also want to assign an appropriate mock survey

Introduction: Managing your mock survey and evaluating your results

Improvement Project Log

Directions: Use this log to help you keep track of all of your improvement projects. Record the names of all of the improvement projects underway, which standards they address, who is responsible for each one, and what the estimated and actual dates of completion are. Once each improvement team has completed its work and determine whether the problem has indeed been solved.

Name of Improvement Project	Addressed Standard(s)	Departments Affected	Team Leader/ Department Manager	Assigned Deadline	Actual Date Completed	Problem Solved? (circle one)
						Yes No
						Yes No
						Yes No
						Yes No
						Yes No
						Yes No

Figure 5

The JCAHO Mock Survey Made Simple, 1999 Edition

team leader to act as the improvement team's liaison and to help ensure it moves in the right direction.

Make sure your improvement teams tackle their assigned project in accordance with the hospital's documented performance improvement (PI) approach. If your teams follow your hospital's chosen performance improvement approach consistently, you may be able to use their results in one of your PI presentations during your actual survey.

Step 7: Follow-up on the success of your improvement projects

As your improvement teams span out across the hospital and take on the task of bringing your hospital into compliance, you'll need to pay close attention to their progress and offer them any help or guidance they may need. Keep a close eye on your list of improvement priorities, and ensure that each problem is being resolved appropriately.

At the same time, you should keep the hospital's department and executive managers up-to-date on the improvement teams' progress. This way, you'll be able to depend on your managers' support if a team gets bogged down by hospital bureaucracy. Encourage the department managers to include a JCAHO preparation update at their regular departmental meetings, as well. This can both help to educate staff on key JCAHO compliance issues and involve them in the survey preparation process.

Pre-Survey Checklist: Accreditation Participation Requirements

The JCAHO requires every hospital to meet certain participation requirements to qualify for and maintain accreditation. A hospital must meet these requirements at the time of its survey, and throughout the three year period until its next survey. There are 10 accreditation participation requirements. You are probably familiar with many, if not all, of them but you might not have thought of them as requirements for participation in the JCAHO survey process. The ORYX requirements (numbers 4, 5, and 6) have been phased in over the last two years. As of January 1, 1999, every hospital is expected to meet all of the ORYX requirements. Review the following statements and the examples to make sure you have all of the requirements in place before your survey. No hospital wants its accreditation in jeopardy over a technicality.

Pre-Survey Checklist: Accreditation Participation Requirements

Requirement	Assessment Point	Yes	No	Example of Compliance	Notes
1	Do you have copies of all of the various licenses, accreditations, and regulatory reports that you have received from any state, local, and national accrediting organizations?	☐	☐	The survey coordinator sends an e-mail to all members of the hospital's executive management requesting that they submit to her copies of the following: all the various licenses, such as the state health department license, the pharmacy license, and the blood gas lab license; all accreditations, such as the CAP accreditation for the lab and the CARF accreditation for the rehab unit; and all regulatory reports, such as the last local health department survey and the OSHA inspection that occurred last year. The survey coordinator then places all copies in a binder.	
2	If your hospital merged, had a significant change in ownership, relocated its plant/facility, or significantly revised its services, did you notify the JCAHO within 30 days of the change?	☐	☐	Your hospital recently merged with another hospital. Your CEO should send a letter to the JCAHO outlining the changes, including how it has impacted your organization and whom the JCAHO may contact for further information.	
3	Have you clearly communicated to anyone who might be in contact with a surveyor that should a JCAHO surveyor arrive unannounced or unscheduled, the surveyor must be allowed to survey the organization, or your accreditation may be jeopardized?	☐	☐	The CEO distributes a policy on handling an unscheduled or unannounced arrival of a surveyor (e.g., a surveyor from the JCAHO, HCFA, the state health department, or another agency) and an administrative all list to all members of management, and reminds managers to communicate to their staffs that there are no conditions under which a JCAHO surveyor would not be allowed to survey the organization.	

Pre-Survey Checklist: Accreditation Participation Requirements

Requirement	Assessment Point	Yes	No	Example of Compliance	Notes
4	Have you verified that • your organization has selected a performance measurement system (from the list of systems that have been approved by the JCAHO) for submitting data to the JCAHO? • you have transmitted your selection to the JCAHO? • any changes in the performance measurement system with which you are participating have been submitted?	☐ ☐ ☐	☐ ☐ ☐	The hospital board has reviewed the list of vendors approved by the JCAHO and, after reviewing several of the programs, has agreed to participate in the Maryland Hospital Association Quality Indicator Project. The hospital has submitted its selection to the JCAHO in writing.	
5 6	Have you verified that • your organization identified and submitted to the JCAHO by January 1, 1998 two indicators that monitor at least 20% of your base population? • one of your indicators measures inpatients? • you began collecting data as of July 1998? • you are submitting monthly data points in your quarterly data? • your performance measurement system is submitting the data to the JCAHO on time? *Note: Your first quarterly report (through your performance measurement system) is due to JCAHO in March 1999.* • your organization has selected two additional indicators, for a total of at least four indicators, that will monitor at least 25% of your base population	☐ ☐ ☐☐☐ ☐ ☐	☐ ☐ ☐☐☐ ☐ ☐	A hospital has chosen its first two indicators as inpatient mortality and returns to the operating room. Because the hospital is using its base population as its inpatient population, inpatient mortality will apply to all inpatients and will monitor 100% of its base population (exceeding the required threshold of 20%). Returns to the OR will apply to the percentage of the population that has surgical procedures. The hospital has selected readmissions within 30 days and post-operative infections as its third and fourth indicators. As with the first two indicators, readmissions within 30 days applies to all inpatients and post-operative infections applies to the number of patients who have had procedures at the hospital. Again, the hospital has exceeded the threshold for all four indicators to monitor, in aggregate, 25% of its base population.	

Pre-Survey Checklist: Accreditation Participation Requirements

Requirement	Assessment Point	Yes	No	Example of Compliance	Notes
cont'd	• you submitted these additional two indicators to the JCAHO as of January 1, 1999?	☐	☐		
	• your performance measurement system is able to submit the data with monthly data points on a quarterly basis?	☐	☐		
	• your organization has a plan to begin collecting your data—with monthly data points—as of July 1, 1999 for your additional two indicators?	☐	☐		
	• your organization has a plan to increase your indicators and base population being monitored as follows:				
	- 2 additional indicators by January 1, 2000, for a total of six indicators that monitor 30% of your base population?	☐	☐		
	- 2 additional indicators, by January 1, 2001, for a total of eight indicators that monitor 35% of your base population?	☐	☐		
	• your organization is able to collect and submit the data for at least four consecutive quarters before you consider changing the indicator?	☐	☐		
7	Do you have a plan to post public notice of your upcoming survey at least 30 days in advance?	☐	☐	A hospital has chosen to serve notice to the public by putting an ad in a local community newsletter and the larger city newspaper and posting large signs at all public and employee entrances to the hospital.	
	Is the notice visible to:				
	• the community your hospital serves?	☐	☐		
	• visitors to your hospital, including patients and families?	☐	☐		
	• all your employees?	☐	☐		

Pre-Survey Checklist: Accreditation Participation Requirements

Requirement	Assessment Point	Yes	No	Example of Compliance	Notes
8	Do you have a plan or a process in place for how you will forward to the JCAHO requests for information concerning your survey? *Note: Make sure you have notified anyone in your hospital who might receive such a request of the appropriate steps to take.*	☐	☐	A hospital has sent a notice to all departments stating that if anyone receives a request for information concerning the upcoming survey, the request is to be forwarded immediately to the survey coordinator's office.	
9	Have you stressed to all who are supplying or preparing information for the survey to not—under any circumstances—alter information or present information that they know to be inaccurate or false?	☐	☐	The hospital does not allow any committee or department to re-write, re-create, or pre-date minutes of any meetings. The hospital verifies that all data and statistics reported to the JCAHO are accurate and consistent.	

Patient Rights and Organization Ethics (RI)

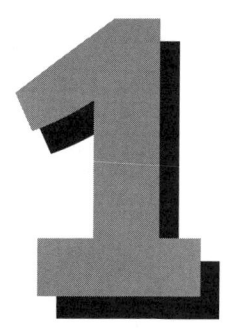

Consumer interest in health care and the popular concept of "the patient as customer" have pushed patient rights and organization ethics (RI) into the spotlight. Ethical decision making has received national attention from the media recently, and consumers want to see that hospitals hold themselves to high standards of integrity at all times, whether the hospital is making decisions about patient care or billing practices.

Recent surveys have shown that a number of institutions continue to have difficulty complying with the patient rights and organization ethics standards. Common problems include:

- involving the patient and family in decisions about the care and treatment of terminally ill patients;
- obtaining consent for blood transfusions; and
- developing an organizational code of ethics.

As you gauge your hospital's compliance with the RI standards, pay close attention to these "hot buttons" and ensure that your organization meets the JCAHO's requirements.

Checklist 1: Patient Rights and Organization Ethics (RI)

Standard	Assessment Point	Yes	No	Example of Compliance	Notes
🏃 RI.1	Does your hospital support a patient's right to: • receive care? • be respected? • understand and participate in all treatment and ethical decisions? • confidentiality and privacy? • select a surrogate decision maker?	☐☐☐ ☐☐	☐☐☐ ☐☐	The hospital's plan of care clarifies the organization's position on patients' rights and requires all employees and medical staff members to treat all patients with respect; staff orientation and continuous training cover the hospital's policy on advance directives and patient confidentiality and privacy.	
RI.1	Do caregivers understand how to address ethical questions?	☐	☐	An ethics committee or team addresses ethical questions; staff orientation and training materials teach caregivers what to do when ethical issues arise; documentation in the medical record describes how an ethical issue was resolved.	
🏃 RI.1.1	Are all patients assured of treatment or service without regard to factors such as: • age? • ethnicity? • ability to pay? • sexual orientation? • a disability?	☐☐☐☐☐	☐☐☐☐☐	Consistent policies and procedures in admitting, the emergency room, ambulatory services, and physician offices all ensure that each patient has equal access to your services; patient information brochures discuss payment options for uninsured patients; aggregate patient data demonstrates that a reasonable patient mix from your given population is served.	
RI.1.1	If you cannot meet a patient's care needs and you must transfer him or her to another facility for treatment, do you: • examine, assess, and stabilize the individual? • ensure that the receiving institution and physician are able to meet the patient's needs?	☐☐	☐☐	A policy ensures the safe and timely transfer of patients who require services the hospital cannot provide, or whose insurance coverage demands treatment at a specific institution. The policy also states that every patient must be assessed, stabilized, and, if necessary, accompanied to the receiving institution once acceptance is confirmed. This is well documented in the medical record.	

The JCAHO Mock Survey Made Simple, 1999 Edition

Checklist 1: Patient Rights and Organization Ethics (RI)

Standard	Assessment Point	Yes	No	Example of Compliance	Notes
✦ RI.1.2 RI.1.2.2 RI.1.2.3 RI.1.2.5 RI.1.2.6 RI.1.2.7	Are patients and their families involved in decisions about their care and treatment, such as deciding: • whether to forgo or withdraw life support? • whether to withhold resuscitative measures? • how to manage pain?	☐☐☐	☐☐☐	A policy requires caregivers to discuss end-of-life decisions with the patient or the patient's representative, respect his or her wishes, and document them in the medical record.	
RI.1.2.1	Do you clearly explain all treatments and procedures to patients and their families, including those that are part of research projects, and obtain patients' written consents for proposed treatments or procedures?	☐	☐	Hospital policy requires physicians to discuss any potential benefits, drawbacks, alternatives, and expected outcomes of all procedures and treatments that carry risk; the hospital's consent manual includes its policy on informed consents and examples of individual consents for specific procedures and treatments; a review of medical records documents compliance with the policy.	
RI.1.2.1	Do all patient consent forms list: • a description of the procedure to be performed? • all potential benefits and drawbacks of the procedure? • any anticipated post-procedure problems? • the procedure's expected success rate? • the expected outcome if treatment is declined? • all reasonable alternatives to the proposed procedure? • the name of the admitting practitioner? • the name of the practitioner performing the procedure?	☐☐ ☐☐ ☐☐☐☐ ☐☐	☐☐ ☐☐ ☐☐☐☐ ☐☐		

Checklist 1: Patient Rights and Organization Ethics (RI)

Standard	Assessment Point	Yes	No	Example of Compliance	Notes
cont'd	• any potential conflict of interest between the practitioner and the hospital or any other related care provider, such as a home infusion company that is co-owned by the physician.	☐	☐		
RI.1.2.1.1 RI.1.2.1.2 RI.1.2.1.3 RI.1.2.1.4 RI.1.2.1.5	Do all patients asked to participate in research projects receive as part of the consent process: • a description of expected benefits? • a description of alternative services that might address their needs? • an explanation of all procedures to be followed? • a clear message that they may refuse to participate without affecting their access to other services?	☐ ☐ ☐ ☐ ☐	☐ ☐ ☐ ☐ ☐	The consent form for all research projects addresses these issues. A review of records of patients participating in research projects identifies compliance.	
RI.1.2.2	Do you involve family members or patient representatives in care decisions as appropriate, particularly in cases where patients are unable to make decisions for themselves?	☐	☐	Medical records note when staff discuss a patient's proposed plan of care with family members; educational materials teach caregivers when and how to involve family members or patient representatives in care decisions.	
♻ RI.1.2.4	Do you ask patients whether they have formulated or would like to formulate advance directives?	☐	☐	A question on the admission sheet prompts admission reps to ask if the patient has an advance directive; a copy of the advance directive is filed in the patient record; a hospital representative aids patients who request advance directives; there is a policy approved by the medical staff addressing advance directives.	

Checklist 1: Patient Rights and Organization Ethics (RI)

Standard	Assessment Point	Yes	No	Example of Compliance	Notes
RI.1.3 RI.1.3.1 RI.1.3.2 RI.1.3.3	Do you protect a patient's right to: • confidentiality?	☐	☐	Your computer system has safeguards to prevent unauthorized access to confidential files. Employees sign an annual acknowledgement of the confidentiality policy.	
RI.1.3.4 RI.1.3.5 RI.1.3.6 RI.1.3.6.1 RI.1.3.6.1.1	• privacy?	☐	☐	Cubicle curtains are used appropriately; waiting areas for gowned patients are separate from general waiting areas; patients are properly covered during transport and bathing. Auditory privacy is also maintained.	
	• security?	☐	☐	Enhanced security measures are taken in the emergency room, the nursery, and pediatrics; security guards are available to protect patients and staff from combative patients.	
	• register complaints?	☐	☐	An organized system exists to receive and address all complaints, whether the complaints are written or verbal, or are received via telephone or in person.	
	• receive pastoral counseling?	☐	☐	Pastoral services are available to patients via an in-house department or a network with community representatives; staff understand how to secure these services for patients.	
	• freely communicate with others to the extent that he or she is able?	☐	☐	Telephone, visitor and all other communication modes are reasonable, based on the patient's condition.	

The JCAHO Mock Survey Made Simple, 1999 Edition

Checklist 1: Patient Rights and Organization Ethics (RI)

Standard	Assessment Point	Yes	No	Example of Compliance	Notes
cont'd	• understand the reasons for any communication restrictions?	☐	☐	Any communication restrictions are fully explained to patients. Limitations are evaluated periodically for necessity and effectiveness.	
RI.1.4	Upon admission, do all patients receive clearly understandable written copies of their rights?	☐	☐	The patient bill of rights is tailored to each patient's age, level of education, and language; this bill of rights is included in the patient handbook or posted prominently throughout the organization; if you have a high non-English-speaking population, your bill or rights is available in translated form	
RI.1.5	Do you obtain protective services, such as guardianship or conservatorship, for patients who require protection?	☐	☐	Cases documented by social services or continuing care indicate when protective services were secured for a patient; the hospital has a mechanism to appoint guardians for mentally incompetent patients.	
RI.1.5	Do you explain to patients how to register a complaint with the state or any other regulatory agency about the quality of care your hospital provides?	☐	☐	The hospital posts a *Medicare Notice to Patients* in all lobbies and waiting areas. The patient handbook includes information on the state department of public health advocacy office.	
RI.2	Has your medical staff developed an organ donation policy or procedure stating: • which organ and tissue agency(s) are affiliated with your organization? • how it will identify potential donors? • who is responsible for approaching the family of a potential donor?	☐ ☐ ☐	☐ ☐ ☐	A contract with a federally approved organ bank is on file; the hospital enforces a policy describing how to identify potential donors and respectfully approach their families; a log is maintained of all potential donors, whether the family accepted or declined the opportunity to donate.	

The JCAHO Mock Survey Made Simple, 1999 Edition

Checklist 1: Patient Rights and Organization Ethics (RI)

Standard	Assessment Point	Yes	No	Example of Compliance	Notes
cont'd	• when and how the family of a potential donor should be approached? • who is responsible for notifying the organ/tissue agency if the family agrees to donate? • when and how to notify the organ/tissue agency if a donation will be made? • how to document the family's consent to donate an organ? • how to document the outcome of the donation? • how to maintain a log of potential donors?	☐ ☐ ☐ ☐ ☐ ☐	☐ ☐ ☐ ☐ ☐ ☐	*Note: In August 1999, the Health Care Financing Administration will begin enforcing recent changes that require notification of all asystolic deaths to the organ/tissue agency.*	
RI.3 RI.3.1	If your hospital conducts research or participates in investigational studies, does it: • safeguard the rights of patients? • obtain informed consents from participating patients? • review each study to ensure that it is consistent with the organization's mission? • gauge the risks and benefits of each study to patients?	☐☐ ☐ ☐ ☐☐	☐☐ ☐ ☐ ☐☐	An institutional review board documents its review and acceptance of each investigational protocol prior to any subject's enrollment.	
🏃 RI.4 RI.4.1 RI.4.2	Does your hospital's code of ethical behavior describe how to handle: • conflicts of interest for board and management? • patient confidentiality? • patients' right of access to services? • billing practices fairly? • marketing and advertising honestly?	☐ ☐☐☐☐	☐ ☐☐☐☐	An ethical behavior policy summarizes the hospital's guiding ethical principles, referencing pertinent policies as needed.	

Checklist 1: Patient Rights and Organization Ethics (RI)

Standard	Assessment Point	Yes	No	Example of Compliance	Notes
RI.4.3	Do you allow patients with long-term stays to perform—or refuse to perform—tasks for the hospital?	☐	☐	A rehabilitation hospital has a program in which patients may copy and collate educational materials, assist in the library, or help maintain the garden. The hospital's ethical code addresses patients' rights to participate in or refuse such tasks, so it is not construed to be free labor for the institution that is against patients' wills.	
RI.4.4	Does the hospital's ethical code address the potential for conflict between clinical decision making and payment to leaders, clinical staff, and licensed independent practitioners.	☐	☐	Medical management policies and documentation in the medical records demonstrate that clinical decision making is based on patients' needs and is not influenced by financial incentives. The hospital's code of ethics clearly states this policy.	

Patient Assessment (PE)

You must have an interdisciplinary assessment process to comply with the patient assessment standards. Disciplines authorized to perform assessments, such as nutrition, rehabilitation, social work, respiratory care, nursing, and medicine, all must prove to surveyors that they work together to thoroughly assess patients and establish an integrated plan of care.

Screening questions that are built into the initial assessment identify the need for dietitians or rehabilitation staff to conduct in-depth assessments. All assessments are available to the health care team on a timely basis to allow integration into the plan of care. Care needs identified through assessment that have not been addressed during the hospitalization are included in the discharge plan. The survey teams will look for an efficient, collaborative, and thorough assessment process that meets the needs of our fast-paced care delivery, either in the inpatient *or* the outpatient setting.

Checklist 2: Patient Assessment (PE)

Standard	Assessment Point	Yes	No	Example of Compliance	Notes
⚑ PE.1 PE.1.1	Are interdisciplinary assessments of the patient's physical, psychological, and social needs: • completed within the time limit specified by your organization? • appropriate to the patient's diagnosis, type of care desired, unit, and history?	☐ ☐	☐ ☐	A medical record review proves that this policy or procedure is followed in all settings; the initial assessment includes screening criteria to identify areas where intensive assessment is needed, such as nutrition.	
⚑ PE.1.2 PE.1.3 PE.1.3.1	Are full nutritional and functional assessments: • performed as dictated by patient needs? • based on criteria applied at initial assessment? Note: All rehab referrals require a complete functional assessment.	☐ ☐	☐ ☐	A dietitian performs a full nutritional assessment when screens in the initial assessment indicate that the patient is at risk for malnutrition or has nutrition needs related to the diagnosis.	
PE.1.4	Are all ordered diagnostic tests • completed in a timely fashion? • available for clinical decision making?	☐ ☐	☐ ☐	Laboratory services maintains a turnaround time of 24 hours or less for routine tests and effectively reports its results.	
PE.1.4 PE.1.4.1	Do your medical records include: • a result for each recorded order? • clinical information that will help clinicians interpret test results?	☐ ☐	☐ ☐	A medical record review proves that this policy or procedure is followed in all settings; each order for a procedure or test results in either a report or an explanation for cancellation. Requests for a CT scan are accompanied by clinical information that justifies the need for the procedure.	
PE.1.5	Do you assess patients' discharge planning needs? Note: This is usually part of the preadmit or admission assessment.	☐	☐	Screening criteria for the admission assessment result in referrals to Social Service/Continuing Care/Case Management for more intensive discharge planning.	

The JCAHO Mock Survey Made Simple, 1999 Edition

Checklist 2: Patient Assessment (PE)

Standard	Assessment Point	Yes	No	Example of Compliance	Notes
PE.1.2.1.1 PE.1.6 PE.1.6.1	Do you require all histories and physicals, nursing assessments, and screening to be: • completed within 24 hours? • available to care providers seven days per week? Note: A history and physical completed within 30 days of admission may be used as long as there is an accompanying note detailing any changes in the patient's status. Medicare requires an update for histories and physicals after seven days.	☐☐	☐☐	Medical records, particularly from weekends and holidays, prove that the hospital process supports availability of information seven days a week.	

PE.1.7
PE.1.7.1
PE.1.7.2
	Do you evaluate all surgical patients to determine whether:
	• they are eligible for surgery or anesthesia?
	• their licensed independent practitioner (LIP) has chosen an appropriate method of anesthesia?
	• an LIP has completed their history and physical within 30 days before planned surgery?
	• the patient's history and physical contains:
	  - a statement of pre-operative diagnosis?
	  - a nursing assessment completed by an RN?
	  - the results of all appropriate tests?
	  - a signed consent form(s), including consent for a transfusion if necessary?
	
	Note: A pre-operative note may be substituted in an emergency, if you have a clear definition, approved by the medical staff, of what constitutes an emergency.
		☐☐
		
		☐
		
		☐☐☐☐
			☐☐
			
			☐
			
			☐☐☐☐
				A policy to "stop the operation" if required information is not on the medical record prior to surgery; caregivers use a pre-surgery checklist to determine whether all required documentation is in the medical record before surgery; interdisciplinary surgical forms note which assessments are required.	

The JCAHO Mock Survey Made Simple, 1999 Edition

Checklist 2: Patient Assessment (PE)

Standard	Assessment Point	Yes	No	Example of Compliance	Notes
🏃 PE.1.7.3	Do you reassess patients immediately before they receive anesthesia?	☐	☐	An anesthesia flow sheet includes a grid for reassessment immediately before induction; the time of the reassessment is noted to establish its relationship to the induction time.	
PE.1.7.4	Do you reassess patients at admission and just prior to discharge from the post-anesthesia care unit?	☐	☐	There is a policy or mechanism to require these critical reassessments at the time of entry and just prior to discharge from the post-anesthesia unit or any site where patients are cared for after anesthesia. A documented review of medical records demonstrates compliance with the requirement.	
PE.1.8	Do you identify and report victims of child, spousal, partner, sexual, and elder abuse?	☐	☐	Criteria to identify potential victims of abuse are available to and understood by all members of the health care team; the social service department is available to consult on potential abuse cases; a policy outlines the hospital's procedure for identifying and reporting abuse.	
	Were all abuse identification criteria developed and approved by appropriate care providers?	☐	☐	Meeting minutes note that an interdisciplinary group, including community representation from the police and agencies, developed all abuse identification criteria.	
PE.1.9 PE.1.9.1 PE.1.9.2 PE.1.9.2.1 PE.1.9.2.2	Are all pathology and clinical laboratory services: • accessible? • provided by an approved hospital lab or reference lab?	☐☐ ☐☐	☐☐ ☐☐	The lab meets stated turn-around times for both stat and routine procedures; the medical staff annually approves a list of federally qualified reference labs; only approved reference labs conduct tests, except in unusual cases.	

The JCAHO Mock Survey Made Simple, 1999 Edition

Checklist 2: Patient Assessment (PE)

Standard	Assessment Point	Yes	No	Example of Compliance	Notes
PE.1.10 PE.1.11 PE.1.12 PE.1.13	Do your waived (point of care) testing policies define: • how waived tests will be performed? • how the results will be used? • who is allowed to perform the tests? • how these individuals must be trained? • how their competency will be tested? • who supervises their performance?	☐☐☐☐☐☐	☐☐☐☐☐☐	Hospital policy allows RNs and patient care techs to perform waived tests that will be used for patient screening and education; waived testing results that are used for treatment decisions are confirmed by the laboratory; waived testing procedures are taught by laboratory personnel.	
PE.1.13	Do staff have access to all waived testing policies?	☐	☐	A full waived testing policy and procedure manual is available on each floor.	
PE.1.14 PE.1.14.1	Do you conduct quality control checks on all testing procedures, such as: • specimen collection and preservation? • instrument calibration? • equipment performance? • test performance?	☐☐☐☐	☐☐☐☐	Laboratory personnel design and monitor quality control activities and unit staff perform them according to laboratory standards.	
PE.1.14.2	Are quality control results saved in a log or file?	☐	☐	A log of quality control results is maintained.	
✺ PE.2 PE.2.1 PE.2.2 PE.2.3 PE.2.4	Do caregivers reassess patients based on: • time elapsed? • response to treatment? • a significant change in the patient's condition or diagnosis? • entry to a new care setting?	☐☐☐ ☐	☐☐☐ ☐	Medical records indicate that patients are reassessed as appropriate.	

Checklist 2: Patient Assessment (PE)

Standard	Assessment Point	Yes	No	Example of Compliance	Notes
🏃 PE.3 PE.3.1	Do you develop and use integrated care plans to help prioritize patient care needs?	☐	☐	Patients' integrated care plans reference all disciplines' findings, note that the hospital takes a coordinated approach to patient care, and are used to prioritize patient care needs.	
PE.4 PE.4.1 PE.4.2 PE.4.3	Do all staff members, including the medical and nursing staff, understand their role in patient assessment and care planning?	☐	☐	The organization's plan of care requires all disciplines to develop patient care plans collaboratively and base them on patients' priorities.	
🏃 PE.5 PE.6 PE.7	Do you specifically assess the needs of: • infants, children, and adolescents? • patients with emotional and behavioral disorders? • patients receiving treatment for substance abuse?	☐☐ ☐☐ ☐	☐☐ ☐☐ ☐	A tailored children's assessment form contains screening criteria appropriate for different age groups and ample room for individualized notes; a special assessment form is used in the addictive disease department.	
PE.8	Do you tailor your assessment to address the special needs of potential victims of abuse?	☐	☐	Prompts on the assessment form, special steps in the assessment procedure, or other mechanisms address the appropriate data collection and sensitivity needed to assess possible victims of abuse.	

Care of the Patient (TX) 3

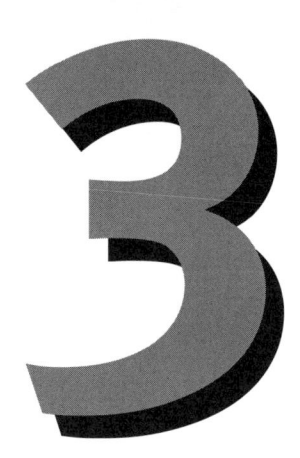

The JCAHO's patient care (TX) standards focus on a wide range of treatment and care issues, such as anesthesia, nutritional, and rehabilitative care and the use of medication, IV conscious sedation, and restraint and seclusion.

As they review your compliance with the TX standards, JCAHO surveyors will expect to see that all departments and disciplines work together to provide patients with excellent care. Often, this form of collaboration is a stumbling block for hospitals since health care workers have historically functioned as separate units. You need to ensure that each person in your organization thinks of himself or herself as a member of a team— a somewhat new concept to many health care disciplines.

In addition, documentation is key in demonstrating your compliance with the TX standards. Many health care workers have trouble finding the time to document their patients' status, and you need to ensure that staff understand how important complete and accurate medical records are to JCAHO surveyors. Documentation must be a top priority—it's really one of the best ways to monitor a patient's progress.

As you review this checklist, evaluate how well your organization demonstrates its compliance with the above two issues, and refer to **Checklist 18: Medical Records, Checklist 20: IV Conscious Sedation vs Anesthesia,** and **Checklist 21: Restraint and Seclusion** for targeted assessment questions for these common problem areas.

Checklist 3: Care of the Patient (TX)

Standard	Assessment Point	Yes	No	Example of Compliance	Notes
☆ TX.1 TX.1.3	Do you regularly review and evaluate the patient's care plan to ensure that it is up-to-date and notes • the results of the patient's initial assessment? • the patient's care goals? • the patient's needs and expectations? • the severity of the patient's illness? • if the patient has any physical or emotional impairments? • if the patient has any disabilities?	☐☐☐☐☐ ☐	☐☐☐☐☐ ☐	A policy states that patient care plans must be reviewed daily to ensure that they are pertinent and address all issues; written care plans are developed at the time of admission by nursing staff, with input from other disciplines as appropriate; these plans are reviewed daily and updated as the patient's status changes.	
TX.1.1	As you set a patient's care goals, do you determine • what services the patient needs? • if the hospital is equipped to provide them?	☐☐	☐☐	The attending physician documents in the admission notes that a patient has chronic renal failure and is on peritoneal dialysis at home and the patient's care plan notes that he or she will require peritoneal dialysis while hospitalized; the hospital is equipped to offer dialysis in the patient's room.	
TX.1.1.1	If you are unable to meet a patient's needs, do you explain why in the medical record?	☐	☐	When a recently diagnosed diabetic who needs to be taught how to deal with his or her illness is admitted to the ICU with multiple trauma, his or her nurse notes in the medical record that diabetic teaching will not be addressed at this time due to the patient's more important life threatening injuries.	
☆ TX.1.2	Do you develop patient care plans collaboratively with • all affected departments? • the patient's family or significant other, when appropriate?	☐☐	☐☐	A stroke patient's care plan should be reviewed by many disciplines, such as physical therapy, occupational therapy, and nutritional care; the nurse reviews the plan for increasing the patient's activities of daily living with the family and encourages them to help care for the patient.	

The JCAHO Mock Survey Made Simple, 1999 Edition

27

Checklist 3: Care of the Patient (TX)

STANDARD	ASSESSMENT POINT	YES	NO	EXAMPLE OF COMPLIANCE	NOTES
🏃 TX.2 TX.2.1 TX.2.2	Prior to a patient's anesthesia induction, do you • assess the patient? • discuss the risks and hazards of anesthesia with the patient and his or her family? • develop an anesthesia plan?	☐☐ ☐	☐☐ ☐	The hospital has a policy for informed consent for anesthesia; medical records note that caregivers discuss anesthesia with patients and their families; anesthesia notes in medical records indicate that patients are reassessed prior to anesthesia induction; a pre-operative checklist prompts caregivers to assess patients before they receive anesthesia; the anesthesia plan is documented in the medical record and made available to all staff.	
TX.2 TX.2.1 TX.2.2	If you offer obstetric or emergency surgery services, do you provide anesthesia within 30 minutes of the documented need for anesthesia?	☐	☐	The hospital and the anesthesia department have a documented policy that requires obstetrical or emergency services patients to receive anesthesia within 30 minutes of their identified need.	
🏃 TX.2.3 TX.2.4 TX.2.4.1	Do you assess anesthesia patients • while anesthesia is administered? • upon their admittance to and discharge from the post-anesthesia care unit (PACU)?	☐☐	☐☐	The anesthesiologist or certified nurse anesthetist documents the results of intra-operative monitoring in the patient's medical record; the nursing staff in the PACU document in the medical record that an assessment was performed when the patient arrived in and was discharged from the unit.	
🏃 TX.3.1	Do you have an inventory of all of the hospital's medications?	☐	☐	The hospital formulary lists each type of medication in the hospital; the formulary was developed by the pharmacy and therapeutics committee and was approved by the medical executive committee.	

Checklist 3: Care of the Patient (TX)

Standard	Assessment Point	Yes	No	Example of Compliance	Notes
TX.3 TX.3.2 TX.3.3	Do you have documented and approved policies and procedures that describe how to safely • order and obtain medications, including those you do not normally stock? • store and handle medications? • control, prepare, and dispense medications?	☐ ☐ ☐	☐ ☐ ☐	The pharmacy, in conjunction with the medical staff and nursing departments, develop policies and procedures describing how to order, store, prepare, and provide patients with medications.	
🥋 TX.3.4	Do you follow all appropriate legal, licensure, regulatory, and professional practice standards and requirements for medication use?	☐	☐	The hospital follows all laws governing the handling of controlled substances and maintains all required documentation.	
TX.3.5	Do you have control mechanisms in place to ensure patient safety when preparing and dispensing medications?	☐	☐	The pharmacist reviews all medication orders for both the correctness and the appropriateness of the medication, dosage, and route of administration. The pharmacist checks for known allergies and other potential drug-drug and drug-food interactions.	
🥋 TX.3.5.1 TX.3.5.5	Do you ensure that medications are • dispensed in an easy-to-administer format? • labeled in a standardized format? • dispensed in sufficient quantities? • available in emergencies or life threatening situations?	☐ ☐ ☐ ☐	☐ ☐ ☐ ☐	The hospital provides nurses with a 24 hour supply of medications, in a single dose form that is easy to identify and dispense.	
🥋 TX.3.5.2	Does a pharmacist review all medication orders, except for those dispensed in an emergency or those not controlled by the pharmacy?	☐	☐	A pharmacist is responsible for reviewing the appropriateness and correctness of all medication orders received in the pharmacy before the order is approved.	

The JCAHO Mock Survey Made Simple, 1999 Edition

Checklist 3: Care of the Patient (TX)

Standard	Assessment Point	Yes	No	Example of Compliance	Notes
TX.3.5.3	Do you distribute patient medication information to all appropriate caregivers?	☐	☐	On admission to the hospital, a nurse documents a patient's known allergies on the patient care plan and on the medication administration record; nursing forwards information on these known allergies to the dietary and pharmacy departments.	
TX.3.5.4	Do you provide pharmacy services 24 hours a day?	☐	☐	A locked medication cart is available to the nursing supervisor when the pharmacy is closed.	
⚹ TX.3.5.6	Do you have a medication recall process?	☐	☐	The pharmacy maintains lot numbers on all medications dispensed by the pharmacy to ensure that in the event of a recall it can retrieve the medication.	
⚹ TX.3.6	Before you give medication to a patient, do you • verify the order? • identify the patient?	☐☐	☐☐	A nursing policy/procedure requires nurses to check all medication orders and each patient's name before medication is administered.	
TX.3.7	Do you allow a patient to self-administer medications brought from home if the physician determines it is medically appropriate to do so?	☐	☐	Patients taking a prescribed non-formulary antacid on a regular basis are allowed to self-administer the medication during their stay in the hospital.	
TX.3.8	Do you monitor the use and disposal of all drugs used in investigational trials or clinical medication studies?	☐	☐	The hospital has policies and procedures describing how to manage investigational drugs; pharmacy records demonstrate that hospital staff properly handle and destroy investigational drugs.	

The JCAHO Mock Survey Made Simple, 1999 Edition

Checklist 3: Care of the Patient (TX)

Standard	Assessment Point	Yes	No	Example of Compliance	Notes
TX.3.9	Do you assess how prescribed medication affects patients?	☐	☐	The nursing department documents the patient's response to medication; the pharmacy reviews each patient's medication profile to ensure that there is no potential for a drug/drug interaction.	
✪ TX.4	Do you screen patients to determine if they are at a nutritional risk?	☐	☐	Caregivers use screening criteria to identify nutritionally at-risk patients, such as patients with cancer and digestive disorders or patients with a history of eating disorders.	
TX.4.1	Do you develop corresponding nutritional therapy plans, if necessary?	☐	☐		
✪ TX.4.2	Before dispensing food or nutritional products, do you require a written diet order from a privileged physician or licensed independent practitioner?	☐	☐	The nutritional services department requires a written diet order from a physician or authorized licensed independent practitioner before it can administer a diet.	
TX.4.3	Have you clearly defined who is responsible for preparing, storing, distributing, and administering food?	☐	☐	Job descriptions and hospital policies and procedures state that the dietary department is responsible for food preparation, food storage, and food distribution, and nursing is responsible for administering food.	
TX.4.4	Do you ensure that meals are • quickly distributed? • the correct temperature? • given to the right patients?	☐☐☐	☐☐☐	The nutritional department requires staff to perform quality checks to ensure that meals are delivered in a timely fashion, to the correct patients, and at the correct temperature.	

The JCAHO Mock Survey Made Simple, 1999 Edition

Checklist 3: Care of the Patient (TX)

Standard	Assessment Point	Yes	No	Example of Compliance	Notes
TX.4.5–TX.4.6	Do you evaluate each patient's dietary intake?	☐	☐	Nursing staff observe their patients' tolerance to their diets and document their observations in the medical record; nursing, dietary, and medical staff use this information to make changes to the diets if needed; the hospital prepares a special diet for patients with lactose intolerance or wheat allergies; the hospital prepares Kosher or vegetarian meals upon a patient's request.	
★ TX.4.7	Are your nutritional care standards • uniformly applied throughout the institution? • developed collaboratively? • readily available in all nursing units and patient care areas?	☐☐☐☐	☐☐☐☐	Diet manuals are developed by the nursing, medical, and dietary staff and are located in all patient care areas.	
★ TX.5–TX.5.1.5	Prior to a procedure, do you note in the medical record the patient's • history? • current physical condition? • potential need for blood?	☐☐☐	☐☐☐	The physician performing the procedure reviews the results of these elements as part of his or her pre-operative assessment.	
★ TX.5.2–TX.5.2.2	Before securing a patient's consent for a procedure, do you discuss • the risks and benefits of the procedure? • if there are any alternative treatments or therapies? • whether blood will be used during the procedure?	☐☐ ☐	☐☐ ☐	The physician discusses the procedure with the patient and his or her family and documents the outcome of this discussion, and the patient's informed consent, in the medical record.	

The JCAHO Mock Survey Made Simple, 1999 Edition

Checklist 3: Care of the Patient (TX)

Standard	Assessment Point	Yes	No	Example of Compliance	Notes
🏃 TX.5.3 TX.5.4	Before and after you perform an operation, do you • evaluate the patient? • develop an appropriate plan of care?	☐ ☐	☐ ☐	According to the pre-operative guidelines developed and approved by the medical staff, the attending physician must document his or her assessment of the patient's mental status, stage of illness, and all relevant, clinical diagnostic criteria; the nursing and medical staff use the data and information gathered during the pre-operative assessment to develop patient care plans.	
🏃 TX.5.3 TX.5.4	Do you monitor each patient's physiologic status during a procedure? Do you document this in the medical record?	☐ ☐	☐ ☐	The circulating nurse documents the patient's status on the intra-operative record; the anesthesiologist monitors the patient's physiologic status during the procedure and documents the results on the anesthesia record.	
🏃 TX.6 TX.6.1 TX.6.2	Are rehabilitation patients treated by qualified, competent staff?	☐	☐	Personnel files and job descriptions note that qualified professionals, such as physical, occupational, recreational, or speech therapists, develop the patients' treatment plans.	
🏃 TX.6 TX.6.1 TX.6.2	Do these qualified individuals develop a written rehabilitation plan, in conjunction with the patient and his or her family, that addresses • the patient's personal rehabilitation goals? • the patient's long-term and short-term rehabilitation goals? • how long it will take to achieve these goals? • what might inhibit goal attainment? • which support systems are available to help the patient meet his or her goals?	☐☐ ☐☐☐	☐☐ ☐☐☐	The rehabilitation plan for a post-stroke patient includes motor and cognitive skill improvement goals and considers the patient's personal goals, emotional state, and access to resources at home and in the community; the hospital develops a special rehab treatment plan for a family of a spinal cord injury patient who wishes to care for the patient in their home.	

The JCAHO Mock Survey Made Simple, 1999 Edition

Checklist 3: Care of the Patient (TX)

Standard	Assessment Point	Yes	No	Example of Compliance	Notes
	• what criteria the patient must meet to achieve greater independence?	☐	☐		
TX.6 TX.6.1 TX.6.2	Does the rehabilitation treatment plan describe what the patient needs to do to reach his or her rehabilitation goals?	☐	☐	The treatment plan for a total hip replacement patient requires the patient to receive acute rehabilitative services twice a day, seven days a week; the hospital has an acute rehab unit which can provide those service as needed.	
TX.6.3	Can you prove that your rehabilitation services help patients?	☐	☐	A review of a patient's rehab treatment plan demonstrates that a therapist frequently measured the patient's progress and adjusted the treatment program, as needed.	
✈ TX.6.4	Do you include written discharge criteria in each patient's rehab treatment plan?	☐	☐	The rehab discharge goals for an elderly patient who lives alone include the ability to • perform activities of daily living without assistance; • stand for five minutes with a walker; • walk 60 feet with a walker.	
	Before you discharge a patient from rehab, do you ensure that he or she has met all treatment goals?	☐	☐	Once the patient achieves all treatment goals, he or she will have met the therapy discharge criteria.	

See ***Checklist 20: IV Conscious Sedation vs. Anesthesia*** for a comprehensive review of these requirements.
See ***Checklist 21: Restraint and Seclusion*** for a comprehensive review of these requirements.

The JCAHO Mock Survey Made Simple, 1999 Edition

Patient and Family Education (PF) 4

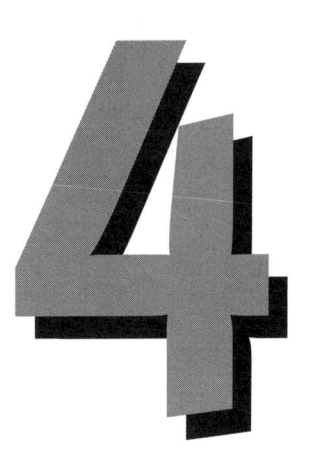

When the Joint Commission's surveyors visit your organization, they will want to find evidence that all departments work together to educate patients and their families, and that caregivers take the time to document how they provide that education. Both of these areas can be weak spots for hospitals. Cross-functional work teams and collaborative planning are still new concepts for many hospital departments, who are used to working as separate entities. In addition, because of downsizing and increased work loads, many caregivers feel pressed for time and find it hard to get around to documenting their educational activities. But, you must remember that multidisciplinary collaboration is key to surveyors and that documentation is your primary means of demonstrating compliance with the patient and family education standards.

Checklist 4: Patient and Family Education (PF)

STANDARD	ASSESSMENT POINT	YES	NO	EXAMPLE OF COMPLIANCE	NOTES
✪ PF.1 PF.1.1	Do you assess each patient's learning needs and determine how they are affected by his or her • culture? • religion? • language? • emotional state? • physical abilities? • motivation? • finances?	☐☐☐☐☐☐☐	☐☐☐☐☐☐☐	Educational plans are structured around any factors that may impact learning. For example, if the patient is blind, provide him or her with educational information in braille, additional verbal instructions, and return demonstrations.	
PF.1.2	Do you identify and educate children and adolescents who require academic schooling while hospitalized?	☐	☐	A policy or plan describes how you identify children or adolescents who need academic education.	
✪ PF.1.3– PF.1.8	Have you developed educational tools to teach patients and their families how to • administer medications safely? • safely use medical equipment? • avoid food and/or drug interactions? • maintain a proper diet? • perform rehabilitative exercises and techniques? • utilize available community resources? • receive follow-up treatment?	☐☐☐☐☐ ☐☐	☐☐☐☐☐ ☐☐	Teaching tools, guidelines, protocols, discharge planning guides, and educational handouts and materials focus on each particular area.	
PF.1.9	Do you explain to patients how they are responsible for their own care?	☐	☐	At the time of admission, patients receive booklets or pamphlets describing the patient and family's responsibilities.	

The JCAHO Mock Survey Made Simple, 1999 Edition

Checklist 4: Patient and Family Education (PF)

Standard	Assessment Point	Yes	No	Example of Compliance	Notes
PF.1.10	Do you have a method to ensure that you meet each patient's personal hygiene and grooming needs?	☐	☐	Each patient is assessed on admission and is reassessed during his or her stay to determine his or her ability to meet his or her personal hygiene and grooming needs. Nursing protocols see that the nursing staff assist the patient as needed in meeting those needs and document that they provided such assistance.	
PF.2	Do you ensure that patients understand what you teach them?	☐	☐	Patients actively participate in learning activities and return demonstrations.	
✈ PF.3	Do you provide the patient, family, extended care facility, or other care organization with instructions describing how to care for the patient after discharge?	☐	☐	Written discharge instructions outline what further care is required, signs and symptoms to look out for, and key phone numbers.	
PF.4 PF.4.1 PF.4.2	Do qualified staff work collaboratively with all departments to educate patients • in an environment where they feel comfortable to ask questions? • with a wide variety of educational tools, programs, and resources that address - patients' needs for specialized instruction? - disabled patients' learning needs? - what community resources are available to help educate patients?	☐ ☐☐☐	☐ ☐☐☐	Educational sessions are unhurried and take place in a private area away from interruptions. The hospital uses an interpreter to help educate deaf patients, or provides booklets or pamphlets in braille and large print for the visually impaired; it refers patients who require specialty programs not offered by the hospital, such as pediatric lipid management, to another organization for treatment.	

The JCAHO Mock Survey Made Simple, 1999 Edition

Continuum of Care (CC)   5

The JCAHO defines continuum of care as the process of matching patients' needs with the appropriate level of care from pre-admission to discharge. This continuum is by no means a new idea for hospitals. Medicare and a number of state agencies have required patient care coordination for years, and many organizations, particularly those in health care networks, have developed far broader definitions of the patient care continuum than the JCAHO's. It's not unusual to find case managers working hand in hand with primary care physicians to manage patients in outpatient or home settings.

If your hospital has a more extensive definition of the patient care continuum than the JCAHO's, or an innovative case management program, surveyors will probably be very interested in learning more about your system. For example, they might focus in on how you identify diagnoses or home situations that require intensive case management or home care to prevent repeated hospital admissions. Surveyors are always on the look out for examples of "best practice" to help them reassess the pertinence of the JCAHO's standards to current practice in the field.

Checklist 5: Continuum of Care (CC)

Standard	Assessment Point	Yes	No	Example of Compliance	Notes
✈ CC.1	Do you ensure that every patient has access to appropriate care?	☐	☐	Mechanisms are in place to assess, and if necessary, stabilize every person who requests treatment, even if the ultimate treatment may be provided by another facility or agency; no patient is turned away due to insurance dictates or lack of insurance.	
CC.1	Are admissions, initial assessments, patient referrals, and transfers handled consistently for all patients throughout the organization?	☐	☐	A medical record review of referred and transferred patient cases verifies that the hospital follows its assessment, referral, and transfer policies and procedures; prior to transfer, a full assessment is performed and documented in the medical record.	
CC.2	Do you ensure that patients receive care in the correct settings by • identifying each patient's individual needs? • determining which area of the hospital can best meet those needs?	☐☐	☐☐	Emergency room patients who require a follow-up visit, have no primary care physician, and have no health insurance are referred to the medical clinic for treatment; a patient admitted to the psychiatric unit is transferred to the neurosurgical floor after an assessment and diagnostic work-up reveals a brain tumor.	
CC.2.1	Have you developed admission criteria for all units and programs in the hospital?	☐	☐	The medical, telemetry, and coronary intensive care units each have quantitative admission criteria that distinguish between the intensity of service provided by each unit; criteria are used to distinguish between inpatients and observation patients.	

The JCAHO Mock Survey Made Simple, 1999 Edition

41

Checklist 5: Continuum of Care (CC)

Standard	Assessment Point	Yes	No	Example of Compliance	Notes
CC.2.1 PE.1	Do you assess patients to determine if they meet the hospital's or the unit's admission criteria?	☐	☐	Assessments elicit the information needed to determine which setting is most appropriate to the patient's needs.	
CC.3	Upon a patient's admission, do you inform his or her family of your plan for the patient's care?	☐	☐	The attending physician or primary nurse speaks with the family and explains the plan of care, expected results, and length of hospitalization; this discussion is documented in the medical record.	
✈ CC.3	Do you ensure that patient and family education occurs upon entry to all settings, including both inpatient and outpatient settings?	☐	☐	When a patient enrolls in a clinic, written information explaining the expected treatment and its potential costs is shared with the patient and family members.	
CC.4 CC.5	As patients are moved in and out of various units, departments, or levels of care throughout their illness, do you coordinate the patient care services they receive?	☐	☐	A case management model ensures that patients receive coordinated care throughout their illness or, alternatively, that all disciplines caring for the patient develop clinical paths collaboratively to ensure continuity of services.	
CC.6	Do you safely discharge, refer, or transfer patients, as needed?	☐	☐	A case management model requires the health care team to develop a safe discharge plan addressing all of the patient's post-discharge needs prior to discharge; transfer agreements exist between your hospital and all rehab, long-term care, skilled nursing facilities, and tertiary care providers normally used by your institution.	

The JCAHO Mock Survey Made Simple, 1999 Edition

Checklist 5: Continuum of Care (CC)

Standard	Assessment Point	Yes	No	Example of Compliance	Notes
CC.6	Do you consider all possible options for post-discharge services?	☐	☐	Home care, adult day care, rehabilitation, home infusion services, outpatient treatment, and placement in a nursing home, either short-term or long-term, are among the options that should be considered for patients who cannot leave the hospital safely without support.	
CC.6.1	Do you update patient assessments just prior to discharge to identify and address any last minute changes in the patient's condition?	☐	☐	Changes in medications, sudden changes in home arrangements, or the patient's willingness to achieve rehabilitation goals should be detected during the patient's reassessment prior to discharge.	
CC.7	Do you share with post-discharge care providers clinical information about your patients, such as • the reason for a patient's discharge, transfer, or referral? • an overview of the patient's health status and the care the hospital has provided? • a list of the community resources offered to the patient?	☐ ☐ ☐	☐ ☐ ☐	Integrated information systems allow for rapid sharing of information as the patient moves within the health care system; discharge summaries and other clinical information, such as the goals of care, medications, diet, physical exercise, follow-up with physician(s), are sent to the accepting care provider; referral forms (required in many states) include all pertinent information needed by the nursing home, rehabilitation facility, home care agency, or other post-hospital care provider.	
CC.8	Do you resolve situations in which the hospital's care team deems that the patient requires treatment not covered by his or her health insurance?	☐	☐	The hospital has a utilization management program that includes an appeal process for denial of health care coverage deemed medically necessary by the attending physician; the appeals process includes a review of the criteria used by the external reviewer and identification of other ways a patient's care needs can be met safely.	

Checklist 5: Continuum of Care (CC)

Standard	Assessment Point	Yes	No	Example of Compliance	Notes
CC.8	Do you have guidelines that spell out how you will work with external reviewers?	☐	☐	The hospital requires language in managed care contracts that describes how external reviewers will interface with hospital care coordination staff and what will happen if there is a dispute over a medical necessity.	

Performance Improvement (PI)

6

The performance improvement (PI) standards are the most important chapter in the JCAHO's *Comprehensive Accreditation Manual for Hospitals.* If you have an organization-wide PI program that weaves PI into the fabric of your organization, you will have no trouble passing your survey with "flying colors." The ideal PI program will

- incorporate JCAHO terminology in your PI plan and all staff educational efforts. This will prevent you from designing a program that is off the mark and will make it much easier for you to demonstrate your compliance to the survey team.
- require everyone in the hospital to use facts, analyze data, and apply statistical process controls.
- require leaders to participate in improvement activities and to understand the link between planning and PI.
- encourage medical staff leaders to get "on board" with PI by participating in a meaningful way.

The 1999 standards allow for more latitude on the part of the hospital, especially in deciding what measures are important for your organization. Continue to include measures focused on monitoring your performance in key processes, high-risk processes, and interventions intended to improve performance.

When your PI efforts become part of your everyday operation, you can rest assured that you will have a successful survey.

Checklist 6: Performance Improvement (PI)

Standard	Assessment Point	Yes	No	Example of Compliance	Notes
PI.1	Do you have an organization-wide approach that is consistently used for • designing new processes? • revising existing processes? • measuring performance? • making decisions about performance? • improving performance?	☐☐☐☐☐	☐☐☐☐☐	Your PI plan explicitly includes all patient care and support services; evidence, such as all staff using the same terminology and approach, indicates that PI is well understood in your organization.	
PI.1.1	Are all PI activities in your hospital performed collaboratively?	☐	☐	Interdisciplinary teams work together on performance improvement projects, and on developing clinical paths and designing new processes; selected performance measures assess the quality of interdepartmental processes. Leaders, medical staff, and employees all use the same approach.	
PI.2 PI.2.1 PI.2.2	As you revise or design new processes, do you ensure that they • are consistent with the hospital's mission and strategic goals? • meet the needs of the customer(s)? • are consistent with current clinical or business practices? • include baseline performance expectations? • consider inherent risks and any published data on the potential for sentinel events?	☐ ☐☐ ☐☐ ☐☐	☐ ☐☐ ☐☐ ☐☐	The hospital uses flow charts, focus groups, and comparative or benchmark data from other providers when developing new processes; pilot testing is used to introduce new processes; pertinent, focused measures test the efficacy of the new process over time.	
PI.3 PI.3.1 PI.3.1.1– PI.3.1.3	Do you systematically collect data • to gauge your current performance? • to measure improvement and document sustained improvement?	☐☐	☐☐	A review of the measures in place for this year provides evidence that you measure important processes to provide assurance that performance is acceptable, that interventions designed to	

The JCAHO Mock Survey Made Simple, 1999 Edition

Checklist 6: Performance Improvement (PI)

Standard	Assessment Point	Yes	No	Example of Compliance	Notes
cont'd	• to identify opportunities for improvement? • on issues identified for more in-depth assessment? • to measure processes with inherent risk?	☐ ☐ ☐	☐ ☐ ☐	improve processes are always documented with measures, that issues that should generate more intensive assessment are measured, and that an occurrence screening program monitors the incidence of processes with risk.	
✈ PI.3.1	Does data collected to gauge performance consider the following: • the selection, patient preparation and education, performance, and post-procedure care for operative and other invasive or non-invasive procedures? • the ordering, administration, and impact of medication use? • the ordering, handling, and administration of blood, and the monitoring of blood use? • the use of restraint and seclusion? • appropriateness of admission, discharges, and transfers? • patient satisfaction? • employee and physician views on performance and performance improvement activities? • behavior management techniques? • risk management activities? • quality control activities? • infection control activities? • other data important to the organization's performance?	☐ ☐ ☐ ☐☐ ☐☐ ☐☐☐☐☐	☐ ☐ ☐ ☐☐ ☐☐ ☐☐☐☐☐	A review of the current organizational measures shows that consideration is given to the scope and complexity of the services you provide, and measures have been selected to reflect this range of services. You can defend the mix and number of measures selected and new measures are added as changes are made to the scope of services. Financial, market share, and other measures that may be required by regulatory or accrediting agencies, are considered in addition to clinical measures.	

Checklist 6: Performance Improvement (PI)

Standard	Assessment Point	Yes	No	Example of Compliance	Notes
☘ PI.4 PI.4.1	Do you systematically aggregate data and assess collected data using run charts, control charts, and other statistical analyses to determine whether a process is stable?	☐	☐	A control chart monitors time to the exam room in the emergency room and demonstrates that for four consecutive days, the time exceeded the upper control limit; assessment of the data showed that out-of-control days were the result of special cause. Aggregated reports on admissions per month by patient unit help leaders make decisions about staffing and bed availability.	
☘ PI.4.2	Do you compare your hospital's performance data against • its own past performance? • recent, relevant references in the current literature? • benchmarks of best practice from other providers? • interactive reference databases?	☐☐ ☐ ☐ ☐	☐☐ ☐ ☐ ☐	Minutes from a planning meeting note that the decision to expand the emergency room was based on data that showed increased waiting times by shift and by day of week compared with the previous year, an increase in patient complaints about delays during the same time period, and a comparison to national data in similarly sized hospitals.	
☘ PI.4.3	Do you conduct intensive assessments • when occurrence reporting identifies a potential or actual sentinel event? • when comparative data indicates a significant variance over time, from other providers or from the literature? • for unacceptable events, such as significant adverse anesthesia incidents, confirmed hemolytic transfusion reactions, pre-op/post-op discrepancies, or significant adverse drug reactions?	☐ ☐ ☐	☐ ☐ ☐	A multidisciplinary team assembles to investigate a potential sentinel event uses analysis tools, such as pareto charts, fishbone diagrams, flow charts, control charts, or others, to determine the root cause(s) of the process failure. After analyzing the data, the team generates recommendations for changes to the process.	

The JCAHO Mock Survey Made Simple, 1999 Edition

Checklist 6: Performance Improvement (PI)

Standard	Assessment Point	Yes	No	Example of Compliance	Notes
⚑ PI.4.4	Do you have a procedure for performing a root-cause analysis that • focuses on identifying system or process problems? • documents recommendations and solutions for problems? • includes a follow-up mechanism to evaluate the effectiveness of your actions?	☐ ☐ ☐	☐ ☐ ☐	A hospital uses the JCAHO format for performing a root-cause analysis. It uses the JCAHO grid (included in a booklet that the JCAHO provides free of charge to all accredited organizations) to record the process. *Note: A hospital may use its own PI model, provided that the hospital analyzes all possible causes, including special and common causes.*	
PI.5	Can you demonstrate systematic performance improvements in your organization over the past 12 months?	☐	☐	PI projects demonstrate that your PI process is effective and measures demonstrate sustained improvement; leaders can describe how significant PI activities fit with the hospital's mission and strategic goals; reports to the governing body summarize significant improvements made within the organization.	

The JCAHO Mock Survey Made Simple, 1999 Edition

Checklist 6: Performance Improvement (PI)

ORYX Questions

1. Have you picked a medical system and 4–8 clinical indicators that represent 25% of your total patient population?

2. Do you have the appropriate hardware and software, if necessary, to meet the requirements of your measurement system?

3. By third quarter 1998, did you begin to collect data on your first set of indicators?

4. Do you have documentation that ensures that the measurement system will submit your data to the JCAHO in a timely fashion?

ORYX Examples

You have selected the Maryland Hospital Association's Quality Indicator Project as your measurement system and have decided to collect data for submission to the JCAHO. You carefully determined that these two indicators meet the 25% requirement. You have selected two indicators for 1998 and two additional indicators for 1999.

The measurement system requires that you have at least a 486 computer and a modem, and have installed the system's software items.

You have reviewed and understand the data requirements for your indicators. You have begun to collect the data in the format specified by the MHAQIP.

Your contract with the measurement system states that the measurement system will submit the data on the selected indicators by the deadline specified by the JCAHO.

Sentinel Events

Note: As of April 1, 1998, the JCAHO asked organizations to self-report certain sentinel events. If you choose to comply with this requirement and minimize the risk of receiving an accreditation watch designation, you might want to consider establishing a policy that addresses sentinel events.

Sentinel Events Questions

1. Do you have a definition of sentinel event that includes:
  - an unexpected event resulting in death or serious injury?
  - an unexpected event that carried the risk of death or serious injury?

Sentinel Events Examples

As part of your policy on sentinel events, include a definition such as: This hospital defines a sentinel event as an unusual, unexpected patient occurrence that results in death or serious injury to the patient; or, in special

Checklist 6: Performance Improvement (PI)

Sentinel Events Questions (cont'd)

2. Do you have a procedure for doing a root cause analysis that:
   - focuses on identifying system or process problems?
   - documents recommendations and solutions to solve problems?
   - includes a follow-up mechanism to evaluate the effectiveness of your actions?

3. Do you have a JCAHO reporting policy regarding sentinel events that requires employees to report:
   - an unexpected event resulting in death or serious injury?
   - abduction of an infant?
   - discharge of an infant to an incorrect family?
   - rape (by an employee or another patient)?
   - a hemolytic transfusion reaction?
   - surgery on the wrong body part or the wrong patient?

   Note: The JCAHO states that a hospital should voluntarily report these events, but does not require reporting. Please check JCAHO literature for full details on the pros and cons of reporting.

Sentinel Events Examples (cont'd)

situations, an event in which the break in process was so egregious that serious injury could have resulted to the patient, posing a threat to other patients if the problem with the process is not corrected.

Use your own PI model, provided you do a thorough analysis of all of the possible causes, including special and common causes, or use the JCAHO format for performing a root cause analysis. *Note: If you choose to use your own PI model, you must put the results in the JCAHO format (see the JCAHO's free booklet about conducting a root cause analysis that was sent to all organizations).*

As part of your hospital policy on sentinel events, include the time frames for reporting, the criteria for inclusion in reporting, the time frames for conducting and reporting a root-cause analysis, and who is responsible to report. For example: The hospital will report within 5 days of the occurrence, or notification of the occurrence, any event that meets the JCAHO reporting criteria (list criteria). A root cause analysis will be submitted within 45 days of notifying the JCAHO of the event. The director of QI/Risk Management will be responsible for determining which events the hospital will report.

Leadership (LD)

7

The leadership standards provide a framework for leaders to establish, maintain, and improve their hospital's patient care services and better meet the needs of their patients and community. While the standards do not require your hospital to follow any particular leadership structure or style, they certainly do describe what the JCAHO expects from the leaders of a "quality" health care organization. Your leaders must prove that they

- ensure that the hospital's services meet the needs of its community;
- establish an atmosphere in which everyone in the hospital effectively communicates and collaborates with each other;
- integrate services for effectiveness and efficiency; and
- support the hospital's performance improvement program.

These standards are extremely important to the overall success of your survey and should be a strong focus of your survey preparation efforts.

Note: The leaders described in the leadership chapter include at least the leaders of the governing body; the chief executive officer and other senior managers; department leaders; the elected and appointed leaders of the medical staff and the clinical departments, and other medical staff members in organizational administrative positions; and the nurse executive and other senior nursing leaders. This definition was clarified in 1998.

Checklist 7: Leadership (LD)

Standard	Assessment Point	Yes	No	Example of Compliance	Notes
❖ LD.1–LD.1.3.2	Do your leaders base all of their operational, strategic, and programmatic plans on your • mission statement? • strategic goals? • vision statement? • values? • community's needs?	☐☐☐☐☐	☐☐☐☐☐	A written plan of care is tied to the needs of your patient population and describes how your services can be accessed by the community; the hospital revises its plan of care to address patient care needs identified through community feedback; the current year's planning document addresses the changes which must be made to meet the hospital's vision.	
LD.1–LD.1.3.2	Does your mission statement outline the purpose of your organization?	☐	☐	The hospital's mission is a succinct statement that clarifies your organization's reason for being.	
LD.1–LD.1.3.2	Do your strategic goals and vision statement • further the hospital's mission? • describe where the organization is headed and how it will get there over the next one to three years? • address identified patient needs?	☐☐☐	☐☐☐	The vision describes what the organization will be in the future; strategic goals are steps the organization expects to take to meet its vision; at least some of your strategic goals are directed at meeting unfulfilled patient needs.	
LD.1–LD.1.3.2	Do the hospital's values identify what is most important to the organization?	☐	☐	Your organization has affirmed its values; these values are guiding principles for the hospital as it works to achieve its mission, vision, and strategic goals.	
LD.1–LD.1.3.2	Are departmental goals aligned with the hospital's mission, vision, strategic goals, and values?	☐	☐	Individual departments should not develop goals that conflict with the hospital's goals; if your organization has just divested itself of psychiatric services, for example, it would be inappropriate for the ambulatory clinic to set a goal to bring in its own psychiatric clinic.	

The JCAHO Mock Survey Made Simple, 1999 Edition

Checklist 7: Leadership (LD)

Standard	Assessment Point	Yes	No	Example of Compliance	Notes
☆ LD.1.1.2 LD.1.1.8	Do all leaders collaboratively make decisions affecting the hospital or your multi-hospital system?	☐	☐	Executive or senior management forums include medical staff leaders as well as senior managers; key planning documents show that leaders work together to identify the need for and design new programs; leaders from all entities in multi-hospital systems meet to establish system-wide policies.	
☆ LD.1.1.3	Have your leaders developed a plan for managing patients under legal or correctional restrictions?	☐	☐	A policy requires all patients to receive appropriate care, despite any visitation, communication, or physical freedom limitations imposed by correctional or legal restrictions.	
LD.1.2	Do leaders ensure that everyone in the hospital is familiar with the hospital's mission, vision, and values?	☐	☐	New employees, volunteers, medical staff members, residents, and agency personnel are familiarized with the hospital's mission, vision, and values during orientation; your mission, vision, and values are topics for discussion at staff meetings and in organization-wide communications.	
☆ LD.1.3.3 LD.1.3.3.1	Do leaders use patient and family satisfaction data to improve your services?	☐	☐	A review of trended, aggregated patient and family satisfaction data gathered over the past three years demonstrates that patient care satisfaction has improved; specific process improvements are linked to a change in patient satisfaction.	
LD.1.3.4 LD.1.3.4.1 LD.1.3.4.2	Do leaders ensure that patients have access to and receive all appropriate services in a timely fashion?	☐	☐	Performance measures indicate that you have acceptable waiting times for important services and acceptable turnaround times for services issuing reports, such as lab or radiology services; policies and procedures require adequate response times to initial requests for services.	

Checklist 7: Leadership (LD)

Standard	Assessment Point	Yes	No	Example of Compliance	Notes
✦ LD.1.4	Have your leaders developed criteria for staff to use to identify performance improvement (PI) priorities?	☐	☐	Prioritization criteria are listed in the hospital-wide PI plan; the PI plan supports on-going identification of improvement priorities; examples of actual improvement activities show how the organization handles priorities set at the beginning of the year as well as flexing to include urgent priorities.	
	Can the priority setting process adjust for unexpected needs?	☐	☐		
LD.1.5– LD.1.5.3	Have your leaders collaboratively developed and gained the governing board's approval of the • annual operating budget? • capital expenditures?	☐ ☐	☐ ☐	As leaders review the budget, they address changes in patient volumes and patient care needs (acuity); reports to senior leadership, medical staff leaders, and/or the governing body update them on the implementation of the budget and capital expenditures throughout the year and explain necessary variances.	
	Were these documents prepared with consideration for patients' care needs?	☐	☐		
LD.1.6	Do leaders require staff to offer all patients the same level of care?	☐	☐	All staff follow consistent patient care policies and procedures, regardless of where a service is performed; medical records indicate that all patients receive the same level of care regardless of setting.	
LD.1.7 LD.1.7.1	Does each department follow an approved, written document that describes its scope of services and goals?	☐	☐	Each department has a document that describes which services it offers, any service limitations, which populations are served, and performance goals.	
LD.1.9 LD.1.9.1	Have your leaders established cohesive staff recruitment, retention, and educational advancement programs?	☐	☐	Low turnover rates, especially in key positions, indicate that employees are satisfied with their jobs; the corporate culture demonstrates that it values employees by offering competitive pay and benefits; a "learning center" offers staff educational opportunities and access to a library.	

The JCAHO Mock Survey Made Simple, 1999 Edition

Checklist 7: Leadership (LD)

Standard	Assessment Point	Yes	No	Example of Compliance	Notes
LD.2–LD.2.10	Are all departments led by designated department directors or managers who are responsible for • ensuring that their departments collaborate with the rest of the hospital? • establishing departmental policies and procedures? • managing their areas' budgets? • improving their departments' performance? • orienting and educating their staff? • making staffing decisions for their areas of responsibility?	☐ ☐ ☐☐☐☐	☐ ☐ ☐☐☐☐	Department managers have up-to-date policies and procedures, appropriate services, well-performing departments, and well-educated staff; managers and medical directors actively participate in information sharing and problem solving forums.	
LD.2.11–LD.2.11.3	Do clinically qualified individuals with clearly defined job descriptions direct your patient care services?	☐	☐	A dietitian is responsible for clinical direction of nutrition services; a physician is responsible for clinical direction in radiation therapy; the physician providing clinical direction in the ambulatory clinic may also be responsible for administrative direction or may share that responsibility with an administrative coordinator.	
LD.3–LD.3.4	Do your leaders ensure that all departments • communicate with each other? • develop policies and procedures with input from all affected departments? • work together to provide patients with the best possible care?	☐☐ ☐	☐☐ ☐	Managers understand how their departments and services interrelate with the rest of the organization; internal newsletters and special bulletins keep managers up-to-date on key projects in the hospital; a new medication administration policy was developed by nursing, the medical staff, the pharmacy, and messenger services.	

The JCAHO Mock Survey Made Simple, 1999 Edition

58

Checklist 7: Leadership (LD)

Standard	Assessment Point	Yes	No	Example of Compliance	Notes
LD.3.3	Do leaders interact with their colleagues at sister health care organizations?	☐	☐	Nursing home and home care agency directors from the same health care network meet to discuss continuum of care issues; planning documents for walk-in services throughout the network assure complete coverage for the population served and avoid duplication of effort.	
🏃 LD.4 LD.4.1 LD.4.2 LD.4.3 LD.4.3.1– LD.4.3.3	Do your leaders support PI in your organization by • studying PI theories and practices? • selecting a single PI approach? • developing a list of processes whose performance must be measured? • receiving information on key measures to gauge organizational improvement and success of improvement activities? • ensuring that these processes are improved, if indicated? • participating in key PI initiatives?	☐☐☐ ☐ ☐ ☐	☐☐☐ ☐ ☐ ☐	Minutes from leadership forums such as management committee, medical executive committee, or governing body meetings indicate that PI is frequently discussed; department directors' job descriptions require them to improve poorly performing processes, and they are evaluated on the success of their efforts; attendance records from PI education programs indicate that all leaders, including key members of the medical staff and governing body, have been trained on PI; minutes of the leadership meetings document appropriate discussion, communication, and actions taken.	
🏃 LD.4.4– LD.4.4.4	Do your leaders support hospital PI activities by • assigning sufficient personnel and time to PI projects? • ensuring that systems are available to support PI activities? • implementing staff training programs on PI?	☐ ☐ ☐	☐ ☐ ☐	Core staff trained on PI serve as a resource for the organization; a budget exists to support staff, the hospital's information systems, and develop training materials; attendance logs indicate that all staff have been trained on PI; hospital information systems are used to aggregate data; minutes from PI team meetings prove that staff have sufficient time to participate in improvement activities.	

The JCAHO Mock Survey Made Simple, 1999 Edition

Checklist 7: Leadership (LD)

Standard	Assessment Point	Yes	No	Example of Compliance	Notes
LD.4.5	Do your leaders evaluate the success of the hospital's PI program?	☐	☐	The quality of the hospital's PI program is evaluated yearly; programs are developed to improve employee participation in the PI program; meetings are held to teach executives how to use PI principles more efficiently in their daily work; employee feedback on the effectiveness of leadership contributions to PI is collected and reviewed.	

Environment of Care (EC)

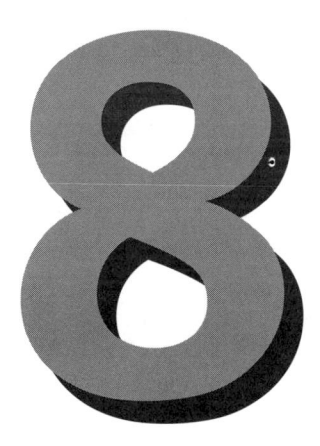

8

The environment of care (EC) standards are a consistent trouble spot for hospitals year after year. In the first six months of 1998 alone, 10 of the JCAHO's top 40 findings were EC-related. Most of these Type I recommendations were given for problems associated with

- the seven required EC plans;
- fire drills;
- equipment and utility preventative maintenance; and
- the *Statement of Conditions™*.

Use this checklist, in conjunction with **Checklist 22: Equipment and Utility Preventative Maintenance** and **Checklist 23: The Seven Environment of Care Plans** to help ensure that your organization is compliant with all of the EC standards.

Checklist 8: Environment of Care (EC)

Standard	Assessment Point	Yes	No	Example of Compliance	Notes
✹ EC.1 EC.1.1	Do all patient care facilities meet the 1997 *Life Safety Code®*?	☐	☐	The hospital's new cancer treatment building constructed in the fall of 1994 meets all life safety requirements.	
✹ EC.1 EC.1.1	Have you completed an up-to-date *Statement of Conditions™ (SOC)* for your organization?	☐	☐	The hospital's *SOC* lists all identified safety problems and describes how they will be corrected; the *SOC* is reviewed and updated at least annually.	
EC.1.2	Do you follow all applicable laws, regulations, and guidelines when you design new space or renovate old space?	☐	☐	When the hospital planned to renovate its pediatric unit, it considered the design recommendations of the Society for Critical Care Medicine, the Centers for Disease Control and Prevention, and the National Fire Prevention Association.	
✹ EC.1.3– EC.1.9 EC.2.2– EC.2.8	Have you addressed the following issues in one comprehensive plan or seven individual management plans: • safety? • security? • hazardous material and wastes? • emergency preparedness? • life safety? • equipment management? • utility management?	☐☐☐☐☐☐☐	☐☐☐☐☐☐☐		

See ***Checklist 23: The Seven Environment of Care Plans*** for specific information on what should be included in each of these plans.

The JCAHO Mock Survey Made Simple, 1999 Edition

Checklist 8: Environment of Care (EC)

Standard	Assessment Point	Yes	No	Example of Compliance	Notes
⚐ EC.2 EC.2.1	Do your employees understand their roles in the hospital's safety program such as • how to initiate the fire alarm? • what to do in case of a fire? • where pull stations, fire extinguishers, and evacuation plans for their work areas are located? • their department's role and their personal responsibilities in an emergency? • how to obtain emergency supplies and equipment? • how to communicate with the rest of the hospital during an emergency? • who to contact in the event of a utility failure? • where utility shut-off valves are located? • where to secure back-up medical equipment? • who to contact in the event of an emergency? • how to contact security in an emergency? • how to minimize personal risk? • how to report a safety or security incident involving a visitor, patient, or employee? • who to contact in the event of a hazardous spill or exposure?	☐ ☐ ☐ ☐ ☐ ☐ ☐ ☐ ☐ ☐ ☐ ☐ ☐ ☐	☐ ☐ ☐ ☐ ☐ ☐ ☐ ☐ ☐ ☐ ☐ ☐ ☐ ☐	All this information should be located in each department's environment of care manual.	
⚐ EC.2.9 EC.2.10	Each year, do you conduct • two emergency preparedness drills, at least four months apart? • fire drills *at least* - quarterly, on all shifts, in patient care areas? - annually, on all shifts, in non-patient care areas?	☐ ☐ ☐	☐ ☐ ☐	Members of the safety committee take turns being observers at each scheduled fire drill. They evaluate how well the drill was conducted by completing a written, criteria-based evaluation that addresses the functioning of the fire alarm system, smoke doors, and the code red team (internal team trained to respond to fire), and the responsiveness of the staff.	

Checklist 8: Environment of Care (EC)

Standard	Assessment Point	Yes	No	Example of Compliance	Notes
cont'd	Do you have a written process fir evaluating whether each fire drill is compliant with your hospital's life safety/safety plan?	☐	☐		
EC.2.9 EC.2.10	If you are a designated emergency center, do you use volunteers to pose as victims?	☐	☐	During a disaster drill for a school bus accident, volunteers posed as the injured school children.	
EC.2.9 EC.2.10	Do you judge whether your emergency preparedness drills and fire drills are effective?	☐	☐	Results of emergency preparedness drills are reviewed and critiqued by the safety committee.	
🏃 EC.2.11	Do you conduct safety inspections or hazard surveillance surveys, at least • every six months in patient care areas? • once a year in non-patient care areas?	☐ ☐☐	☐ ☐☐	Safety committee members take turns inspecting various areas of the hospital using a safety assessment tool; this tool prompts users to evaluate basic safety items such as fire doors, pull stations, and doorways.	
EC.2.11	Have you defined • how often you will perform safety inspections? • who will perform the inspections? • how the results of the inspections will be reported? • how you will address identified deficiencies?	☐ ☐☐ ☐	☐ ☐☐ ☐	The safety committee has developed a policy describing how safety inspections should be performed.	
See ***Checklist 22: Equipment and Utility Preventative Maintenance*** for a comprehensive review of preventative maintenance requirements.					

The JCAHO Mock Survey Made Simple, 1999 Edition

Checklist 8: Environment of Care (EC)

Standard	Assessment Point	Yes	No	Example of Compliance	Notes
EC.3	Do you collect data and information on the status of your hospital's safety, security, hazardous materials and wastes, emergency preparedness, life safety, and equipment and utility management programs?	☐	☐		
EC.3	Do you use this information to identify improvement opportunities?	☐	☐	The hospital uses performance standards and indicators to help monitor the hospital's compliance with each of the seven safety programs; the safety committee reviews this data and identifies opportunities for improvement.	
EC.3.1	Is someone in your hospital designated to manage the hospital's safety program?	☐	☐	The hospital has a safety director who oversees all components of the safety program.	
EC.3.2	Does your hospital have a safety committee who reviews and evaluates safety issues and recommends to administration at least one performance improvement activity per year?	☐	☐	The hospital's safety committee is comprised of representatives from the laboratory, plant operations, infection control, nursing, quality improvement, risk management, administration, radiology departments; these individuals meet monthly to discuss hospital safety issues and to review ongoing monitoring activities for each of the seven safety programs. After reviewing these monitoring activities, the committee makes recommendations for PI projects to administration.	
EC.4– EC.4.4.2	Do you provide each patient with appropriately furnished, private space that is safe, comfortable, and clean?	☐	☐		

The JCAHO Mock Survey Made Simple, 1999 Edition

Checklist 8: Environment of Care (EC)

Standard	Assessment Point	Yes	No	Example of Compliance	Notes
cont'd	Do you ensure that each patient room has adequate lighting and ventilation?	☐	☐		
	Do you offer each patient space to store personal items?	☐	☐		
	Do you help patients with their personal hygiene and grooming, if necessary?	☐	☐		
	Do you allow patients to wear their own clothing, if possible?	☐	☐		
	Do you give each patient access to a telephone?	☐	☐		
	Do you allow patients to participate in outdoor activities if their conditions permit?	☐	☐		
	Do all locked spaces meet the requirements of the 1997 *Life Safety Code®*?	☐	☐		
	Do you have access to all locked spaces during emergencies?	☐	☐		
	Do you provide for patient privacy?	☐	☐		
	Do you house no more than eight patients in one room (except under special circumstances)?	☐	☐		

Checklist 8: Environment of Care (EC)

Standard	Assessment Point	Yes	No	Example of Compliance	Notes
cont'd	If a patient is hospitalized for a long period of time, do you provide opportunities for social interaction if he or she desires and if it is clinically appropriate?	☐	☐		
	Do you provide furnishings and equipment that is age-specific, meets the needs of disabled patients, and provides for clinical/therapeutic needs?	☐	☐		
🏃 EC.5 EC.5.1	Do you have a written "No Smoking" policy that's stringently enforced?	☐	☐		
EC.5 EC.5.1	Before a patient can be excepted from the no smoking policy, do you • decide whether he or she meets the "exception criteria?" • secure a physician order allowing the patient to smoke?	☐ ☐	☐ ☐		
EC.5 EC.5.1	Do you have a "smoking area" for patients excepted from the no smoking policy?	☐	☐	The hospital has a well ventilated patient smoking room.	
EC.5 EC.5.1	Does it have adequate airflow and circulation?	☐	☐		
EC.5 EC.5.1	Do you have designated employee smoking areas located away from the hospital's entrances?	☐	☐	The hospital has a designated employee smoking area, complete with ashtrays and benches, outside the employee entrance.	

The JCAHO Mock Survey Made Simple, 1999 Edition

Human Resources (HR)

The human resources (HR) standards require hospitals to maintain a competent and adequate number of staff at all times. This may seem to be an easy task on the surface, but in truth over 20% of the hospitals surveyed during the first half of 1998 received a Type I recommendation for competence assessment (HR.5), and many other hospitals failed to meet surveyors' expectations for collection, aggregation, and reporting of staff competence data (HR.4.3).

Keep these two trouble spots in mind as you conduct your mock survey. Ensure that your competency assessments are critical to each person's job performance and relevant to the types and ages of the patients each staff member serves. In addition, you should review your annual HR report to the board of directors to verify that you consistently report staff performance evaluation data to the board of directors.

Checklist 9: Human Resources (HR)

Standard	Assessment Point	Yes	No	Example of Compliance	Notes
HR.1	Have you identified and defined the requirements, duties, and goals for each position in your organization?	☐	☐	Written job descriptions are on file for each position in your hospital.	
✣ HR.1	Do you have criteria-based job descriptions for each position in your organization?	☐	☐	Written job descriptions include objective, written, performance-based criteria that is used to evaluate each employee's performance.	
HR.1	Do leaders compare staff capabilities and competencies with staffing needs to determine whether current staffing levels are appropriate?	☐	☐	A review of staffing plans demonstrates that the hospital lacks a sufficient number of physical therapists. In response, a physical therapist recruitment program is developed.	
HR.2	Do you have an adequate number of appropriate, qualified, and trained employees?	☐	☐	Each department's staffing plan shows how it accommodates increases and decreases in work loads using on-call staff or part-time staff.	
HR.2	Do you to adjust staffing levels to meet departmental needs?	☐	☐	Master staffing plans for the operating room include suggestions on how best to increase and decrease staffing levels; the operating room maintains a call roster and a list of cross-trained employees—e.g., the nurse manager of the OR—who can circulate in the OR if necessary.	
✣ HR.2	Do you verify that all employees, as appropriate, meet regulatory, licensing, and legal requirements for • education and training? • experience and competence? • licensing, certification, registration?	☐☐☐	☐☐☐	The human resources department validates each job candidate's education and training, previous employment, and current license, registration, and/or certification.	

The JCAHO Mock Survey Made Simple, 1999 Edition

Checklist 9: Human Resources (HR)

STANDARD	ASSESSMENT POINT	YES	NO	EXAMPLE OF COMPLIANCE	NOTES
❉ HR.3	Do you evaluate and measure the competence of all employees, including contracted employees, on a regular basis?	☐	☐	Documentation indicates that the hospital uses criteria-based annual performance appraisals and competence assessment tools to evaluate employee competence.	
❉ HR.3	Do you improve employee competence by educating and training staff?	☐	☐	Orientation and training on specialized equipment maintains employee competence.	
HR.3.1	Do you assess staff development needs on a • hospital-wide basis? • departmental basis? • individual basis?	☐☐☐	☐☐☐	The hospital's education department uses surveys, such as written needs assessments, to identify employees' educational and training needs.	
HR.3.1	Do you use the results of these staff development assessments to create staff education plans?	☐	☐	A hospital-wide needs assessment of all employees reveals that many individuals do not know how to handle a chemical spill. As a result, the educational department presents an educational program, open to all interested employees, on how to handle hazardous materials.	
HR.3.1	Do you encourage employee growth and development?	☐	☐	Your education department offers internal and external continuing education programs, such as patient fall prevention and fire safety programs.	
❉ HR.4 HR.4.1	Do you have an employee and volunteer staff orientation program that teaches staff how to safely and competently perform their duties?	☐	☐	General hospital and department specific orientation programs are offered to all new staff.	

The JCAHO Mock Survey Made Simple, 1999 Edition

Checklist 9: Human Resources (HR)

Standard	Assessment Point	Yes	No	Example of Compliance	Notes
🏃 HR.4 HR.4.1	Do you educate staff on • general patient, employee, and volunteer safety? • infection control and employee health? • the hospital's values, mission, and vision? • the hospital's performance improvement program? • important issues related to their new department?	☐☐☐☐ ☐	☐☐☐☐ ☐	The orientation curriculum for new employees covers • fire safety, hazardous materials policies; • universal precautions, personal protective equipment; • the hospital's mission, vision, and values; and • performance improvement. New employees are oriented to • the location and use of MSDS; and • departmental policies and procedures.	
HR.4.1	Do you orient forensic staff, correctional officers, and guards to • hospital and departmental reporting structures and lines of communication? • proper use of restraint/seclusion as it relates to the forensic staff's job? • the hospital's emergency call system? • the procedure for reporting incidents or unusual occurrences?	☐ ☐ ☐ ☐	☐ ☐ ☐ ☐	The hospital provides county police officers who guard patients in the emergency department; staff are taught how to properly use restraint and seclusion.	
HR.4.2	Do you hold inservices and other educational sessions to • improve overall staff competence? • ensure that employees understand how to use new equipment? • teach employees how to comply with new procedures?	☐ ☐ ☐	☐ ☐ ☐	Staff development programs are held on issues such as restraint or seclusion. Orientation and training programs are held for all employees who will operate new equipment. Records indicate that the hospital taught employees how to operate a new peritoneal dialysis machine.	

The JCAHO Mock Survey Made Simple, 1999 Edition

Checklist 9: Human Resources (HR)

Standard	Assessment Point	Yes	No	Example of Compliance	Notes
HR.4.2	Do you periodically assess employee job performance?	☐	☐	Annual performance appraisals and competence assessments.	
🏃 HR.4.3	Is data on staff competence • collected and analyzed for patterns, trends, and opportunities for improvement? • used to identify areas where additional staff education and training is needed? • reported annually to the hospital board of directors?	☐ ☐ ☐	☐ ☐ ☐	Aggregate results from performance appraisals and/or competence assessments note a weakness in customer service, and therefore an inservice program is developed to strengthen this area.	
🏃 HR.5	Do you periodically assess and evaluate all employees' abilities to perform their jobs and meet the age-specific and other special needs of the populations they serve?	☐	☐	Competency assessment tools are used to evaluate whether staff are qualified to provide care to elderly patients.	
HR.5	Have you identified the different age and other special needs groups in the populations your hospital serves?	☐	☐	A review of historical demographic data obtained at admission indicates which areas of your hospital serve which types of patients.	
🏃 HR.6 HR.6.1 HR.6.2	Do you have a policy or procedure readily available to all employees which • identifies which care situations might conflict with a staff member's cultural, ethical, or religious beliefs? • gives employees the right to request not to participate in a care situation because of their beliefs? • describes the process you will follow to ensure that patient care is not jeopardized should you grant this request?	☐ ☐ ☐	☐ ☐ ☐	Your policy states that temporary agency staff or on-call staff may be brought in to handle a case that conflicts with a caregiver's beliefs until the employee can be reassigned to another area.	

The JCAHO Mock Survey Made Simple, 1999 Edition

Information Management (IM) 10

The JCAHO's information management (IM) standards set requirements for the hospital's health information management (medical records), medical library, and information systems.

Many organizations focus all of their efforts on gauging how well their information systems capture and synthesize data, and spend little time reviewing their medical records or the quality of their library's resources. Don't let your organization fall into this trap. All of the IM standards are important, and many hospitals receive JCAHO Type I findings in the areas of medical record completion, authentication of orders, and documentation of operative notes. (See **Checklist 18: Medical Records** for a complete listing of all of the components that should be included in your medical records.)

You can also expect your survey team to closely review your information plan to ensure that it is appropriate for your scope of services and was developed collaboratively. If your information services department develops your information plan alone, it will not pass muster. Surveyors expect to see that all of your IM processes are developed with multidisciplinary input.

Checklist 10: Information Management (IM)

STANDARD	ASSESSMENT POINT	YES	NO	EXAMPLE OF COMPLIANCE	NOTES
🏃 IM.1	Do you have an information management (IM) plan that describes how the organization will address its information needs?	☐	☐	The plan describes how the hospital will address its information needs through an interdisciplinary steering committee.	

🏃 IM.1	Does the plan specifically address:
	• the hospital's size, scope, and complexity?
	• customers' information needs?
	• the hospital's information needs for:
	  - planning?
	  - research?
	  - education?
	  - reporting?
	  - data transmission?
	  - performance improvement (PI)?
	  - customer-supplier relationships?
	  - data comparisons and benchmarking?
	  - decision and resource consumption analysis?
	  - improving work flow?
	  - historical and longitudinal reporting?
	  - meeting relevant national guidelines for data set parity and data connectivity?
	  - appropriate technology, such as need for increased storage, use of laptops by users throughout the system, or scanning devices for tracking efficiency?
	• the cost and cost-effectiveness of implementing the plan?
	• how it will support clinical and administrative decision-making?
		☐☐ ☐☐☐☐☐☐☐☐ ☐☐☐ ☐ ☐ ☐	☐☐ ☐☐☐☐☐☐☐☐ ☐☐☐ ☐ ☐ ☐	The plan was developed with input from a multidisciplinary steering committee and was approved by hospital leadership; the plan is reviewed and updated informally at the quarterly meetings of the steering committee and formally updated annually; the capital expenditure process reflects the acquisitions required by the plan.	

The JCAHO Mock Survey Made Simple, 1999 Edition   77

Checklist 10: Information Management (IM)

Standard	Assessment Point	Yes	No	Example of Compliance	Notes
cont'd	• any plans to expand or revise computer services, medical records, or library services? • any long-range plans likely to affect the hospital's information needs?	☐ ☐	☐ ☐		
IM.1.1 IM.1.1.1	Does the hospital have adequate processes, staff, and resources to efficiently run its • medical records department? • information services department • medical library?	☐☐☐	☐☐☐	The hospital can demonstrate that it does not suffer from information systems failures, such as the transcription system being down and a frequently closed library.	
🥋 IM.1.1.2	Was your IM plan developed with input from all affected areas of the organization, both clinical and administrative?	☐	☐	Minutes of appropriate forums, such as a steering committee, indicate that leaders discuss what should be included in the IM plan.	
🥋 IM.2 IM.2.1 IM.2.3	Do you ensure that data and information are confidential, secure, and accurate?	☐	☐	Employee orientations, staff meetings, and training sessions focus on the importance of information confidentiality; the human resources department has a policy stating that breaches of confidentiality are immediate grounds for dismissal; information systems are guarded with passwords which are changed every three months.	
IM.2 IM.2.1 IM.2.3	Have you established who is allowed to access medical records and other information in the hospital?	☐	☐	If passwords are used, they are deleted from the system when employees leave; if you allow physicians to "call-in" to your computer system, you verify that the caller should have access, perhaps by requiring the user to enter a patient record number; highly sensitive portions of the medical record are kept in a separate location.	

Checklist 10: Information Management (IM)

Standard	Assessment Point	Yes	No	Example of Compliance	Notes
IM.2–IM.2.3	Does the health information department only release medical records to comply with a subpoena, court order, or statute?	☐	☐	The hospital has clearly defined, in accordance with state and federal regulations, when and to whom a medical record may be released.	
IM.2.2	Do your systems for collection, storage, and retrieval of data support the timely and easy use of data, without breaching confidentiality and security requirements?	☐	☐	Surveys of MDs and RNs demonstrate that the systems meet the needs of MDs and RNs for timely availability of patient care data. Tracking on hospital information systems demonstrates that appropriate personnel access data. Employee interviews demonstrate knowledge of policies and procedures for access.	
IM.2.3	Do you protect your information system and medical records from disasters, such as a fire?	☐	☐	Sprinkler or Halon systems protect medical records; there is a disaster recovery program for information systems.	
IM.3–IM.3.2	Is data gathered and maintained systematically using • uniform data definitions and data capture methods? • minimum data sets? • codes and classifications?	☐ ☐ ☐	☐ ☐ ☐	The medical records department utilizes the ICD-9-CM coding system as well as the CPT coding system as required by payors; the library utilizes the National Library of Medicine Classification System; the nursing division adheres to the North American Nursing Diagnoses Association List of Approved Diagnoses.	
IM.3–IM.3.2	Has the health information management department defined how data should be gathered for various purposes, such as • ICD-9-CM? • CPT? • SNOMED?	☐ ☐ ☐	☐ ☐ ☐	Required data are defined and captured systematically.	

The JCAHO Mock Survey Made Simple, 1999 Edition

Checklist 10: Information Management (IM)

Standard	Assessment Point	Yes	No	Example of Compliance	Notes
cont'd	• state requirements for birth or cancer registration?	☐	☐		
IM.3– IM.3.2	Do you have an approved abbreviation list that is updated annually?	☐	☐	All abbreviations used in the medical record are catalogued, reviewed, and approved annually; all hospital staff who work with the medical record understand how to interpret each abbreviation correctly.	
IM.3– IM.3.2	Are there uniform reporting and search tools in use in the medical library?	☐	☐	The library uses Medical Subject Headings (MESH) for searches; forms used to request MESH searches are available in the library.	
IM.3– IM.3.2	Is data gathered quickly and efficiently?	☐	☐	Current reports are readily available to staff to help them make patient care decisions.	
IM.3.2.1	Does your organization conduct continuous review of the quality and timeliness of medical records?	☐	☐	Results of one of the following types of reviews are folded into the performance improvement program to establish a level of performance and identify information management issues for improvement: • Representatives of all disciplines on the care team conduct concurrent review of records for required elements. The review is on a rotating calendar, i.e. full record review for ambulatory care in January, Medical Floor in February, Outpatient Surgery in March. **or** • Staff at all care sites conduct focused reviews on a scheduled basis, (e.g. in January, all sites review records for compliance with	

The JCAHO Mock Survey Made Simple, 1999 Edition

Checklist 10: Information Management (IM)

Standard	Assessment Point	Yes	No	Example of Compliance	Notes
cont'd				assessment requirements; in February, all sites review records for compliance with advance directive requirements; in March, all sites review discharge requirements; etc.)	
IM.3.2.1–IM.3.2.1.2	Do you communicate the results of your medical record reviews?	☐	☐	Minutes from the medical record committee or medical executive committee documenting the results of medical records reviews are communicated to leaders; identified issues are forwarded to the appropriate chiefs of service and vice presidents.	
See ***Checklist 19: Medical Records*** for a complete listing of each item that should be documented in the medical record.
IM.4	Do you educate your leaders and staff on how to manage the hospital's information?	☐	☐	Continuing education records demonstrate that staff and leaders have been educated on IM; attendance logs indicate that appropriate staff have been taught how to use the hospital's information system; the results of employee surveys prove that IM education is directed at identified educational needs.	
IM.5 IM.5.1	Is your data and information transmitted to users quickly and efficiently?	☐	☐	The lab's computer system interfaces with the hospital-wide information system; reliable dictation or FAX systems speed data transmission in organizations without an information system; the pharmacy receives orders through the FAX.	

The JCAHO Mock Survey Made Simple, 1999 Edition

Checklist 10: Information Management (IM)

Standard	Assessment Point	Yes	No	Example of Compliance	Notes
IM.5–IM.5.1	Do you minimize data and information transmission errors?	☐	☐	The hospital uses checks to help minimize errors and identify data entry errors, such as ensuring that dosages on drug orders are reasonable or automatically delta checking lab results.	
IM.6	Do you integrate and interpret gathered information?	☐	☐	The hospital combines clinical and financial information into meaningful reports for decision making; system documentation proves that you follow HL7 standards for integrating your information with other systems, such as reference databases.	
IM.6.1	Have you stipulated in accordance with state and federal guidelines how long medical records can be stored and how that information may be used?	☐	☐	The full medical record is stored for 30 years (or whatever your state requires) in a secure area with appropriate climate control; a lifetime medical record, with agreed upon components from the full medical record, is placed for on-line use in integrated care delivery systems.	
IM.7–IM.7.2	Do you appropriately manage patient data and information by defining • what information should be included in the medical record? • who is authorized to make entries in the medical record?	☐ ☐	☐ ☐	Medical record policies stipulate which disciplines are responsible for updating which components of the record; unauthorized entries to the medical record, including data from unknown sources, are not accepted.	

The JCAHO Mock Survey Made Simple, 1999 Edition

Checklist 10: Information Management (IM)

Standard	Assessment Point	Yes	No	Example of Compliance	Notes
IM.7–IM.7.2	Does the hospital establish a medical record for every patient who receives care and treatment?	☐	☐	Each new patient receiving care or treatment is issued a medical record number; the hospital does not create a medical record only for performed diagnostic tests—instead it retains the record of the procedure in the departmental records in accordance with state and federal regulations.	
IM.7–IM.7.2	Does each medical record provide the information necessary to care for the patient in the next setting or by other care providers in the current setting?	☐	☐	The medical record should have all the information any qualified care provider will need to continue a patient's care and treatment if the current provider is suddenly unavailable; hospital standards require all records to include all necessary clinical and demographic information, such as the patient's history and physical, assessment, medications, laboratory and imaging results, treatments, and discharge summary.	
☼ IM.7.4 IM.7.4.1	Do you generate a problem list for every ambulatory patient who visits a clinic three or more times? *Note: Highly focused ambulatory services may be excluded from this requirement if hospital policy defines this exclusion.*	☐	☐	Medical record policies and medical staff regulations require problem lists to be included in specified ambulatory records; the problem list describes all significant diagnoses and procedures, medications, and allergies; the list is reviewed and updated as necessary at each visit.	
IM.7.4 IM.7.4.1	Do you share problem lists with other outpatient settings if records are kept separately?	☐	☐	The hospital includes all problem lists on the hospital information system (HIS) so all care providers can access them; manual record retrieval systems are efficient when no HIS exists.	

The JCAHO Mock Survey Made Simple, 1999 Edition

Checklist 10: Information Management (IM)

Standard	Assessment Point	Yes	No	Example of Compliance	Notes
IM.7.5–IM.7.5.3	Do your medical records contain the following when emergent, urgent, or immediate care is provided? • time and means of arrival? • conclusions, condition at discharge, final disposition, and instructions for further care? • a note if the patient left against medical advice? Is there a mechanism for providing a copy of the medical record to the practitioner responsible for follow-up care?	☐ ☐ ☐ ☐ ☐	☐ ☐ ☐ ☐ ☐	Hospital policy requires these elements in the medical record and a review of medical records for patients of this type demonstrates 100% compliance.	
IM.7.3–IM.7.3.1	Do your records contain a pre-operative or pre-procedure diagnosis for all patients?	☐	☐	The history and physical or short form assessment includes the pre-procedure diagnosis in 100% of records reviewed.	
IM.7.3.2–IM.7.3.2.2	As soon as possible after surgery, are operative notes • dictated or written? • transcribed? • authenticated by the responsible practitioner? • included in the medical record?	☐ ☐ ☐ ☐	☐ ☐ ☐ ☐	The hospital has a medical staff policy, supported by surgical leadership, that requires surgeons to write at least a hand-written operative note immediately after surgery and have the full note transcribed and added to the patient's chart within 24 hours of the completion of the procedure.	
IM.7.3.3	Is there detailed documentation of the patient's post-procedure course—including vital signs, fluids, and blood—as well as management of any post-operative events?			The progress notes, a special flow sheet, or some other mechanism details the patient's post-procedure course in 100% of the medical records reviewed.	

Checklist 10: Information Management (IM)

Standard	Assessment Point	Yes	No	Example of Compliance	Notes
IM.7.3.4	Can you demonstrate that every patient meets criteria for discharge from the post-anesthesia care unit?	☐	☐	A flow sheet, physician order sheet, clinical path, or some other mechanism documents that each patient met criteria for discharge from the post-anesthesia care unit.	
IM.7.3.5	Do your records clearly show the name of the licensed independent practitioner who was responsible for discharging the patient from the post-anesthesia care unit?	☐	☐	A review of medical records demonstrates that the name of the discharging practitioner was recorded 100% of the time. In organizations which have a robust information system that is networked to MD offices, the follow-up information may be accessible online.	
⊛ IM.7.6	Are all of your medical records completed within 30 days of discharge? Is your volume of delinquent records less than 50% of the average monthly discharges for each of the last four quarters?	☐ ☐	☐ ☐	All physicians have equal access to the medical record following patient discharge; the hospital has a physician-friendly record completion process, with positive incentives for prompt completion; you have a system to monitor record completion; chiefs of service are made aware of delinquency rates in their areas.	
⊛ IM.7.7	Do the medical staff rules and regulations stipulate who can receive and transcribe verbal orders?	☐	☐	Medical staff rules and regulations allow RNs and RPhs to receive and transcribe verbal orders.	
⊛ IM.7.8	Are all entries in the medical record • dated, timed, identified by author and, if necessary, authenticated?	☐	☐	The discharge summary, operative report, history and physical report, and all consultations are signed and dated by the appropriate individuals.	

The JCAHO Mock Survey Made Simple, 1999 Edition

Checklist 10: Information Management (IM)

Standard	Assessment Point	Yes	No	Example of Compliance	Notes
cont'd	• made by authorized individuals?	☐	☐	All orders on the physician order sheet are either written and signed by a physician, or written by an authorized individual and authenticated later by a physician.	
★ IM.7.7	Have you defined which telephone and verbal orders must be authenticated within a specified time period?	☐	☐	The medical staff has defined those orders which they agree cannot be given verbally and must be authenticated within a specified time period, such as those for restraint, medication use, and invasive procedures; the hospital requires restraint orders to be authenticated within one hour and all other orders to be authenticated within eight hours.	
IM.7.9	Does your organization have a mechanism that allows for all relevant components of a medical record to be assembled when the patient requires care in the emergency department or an ambulatory setting?	☐	☐	The medical staff has identified and approved those elements of the medical record that are considered vital for patient care and there is a mechanism in place to make sure this information is available 24 hours a day, seven days a week, including holidays. The mechanism can be manual (a position on each shift with responsibility to do this) or electronic (centralized information system that holds this information for each patient seen in the organization, regardless of site).	
IM.8	Do you review aggregated data?	☐	☐	Reports based on aggregated data are used to support patient care, decision making, management and operations, trend analysis, performance comparisons, and PI.	

The JCAHO Mock Survey Made Simple, 1999 Edition

Checklist 10: Information Management (IM)

Standard	Assessment Point	Yes	No	Example of Compliance	Notes
IM.9– IM.9.2	Do you make clinical literature available to staff?	☐	☐	An on-site medical library offers accurate, current literature and periodicals, search capabilities to access databases of information not available on site; meeting minutes and planning documents indicate that the quality of the hospital's clinical resources are assessed.	
🏃 IM.10– IM.10.3	Do you compare your hospital's data with other organizations' data?			Written agreements indicate that the hospital participates in benchmarking programs such as the Maryland Hospital Association's comparative database, a state-required database, a cancer registry, or any other reference database; minutes from PI team meetings indicate that the comparison data is discussed; the hospital's IM plan addresses the need to compare data and information with outside sources. *Note: JCAHO has established a list of approved comparative databases. These should be considered as you make future plans for comparative activities.*	

Infection Control (IC)   11

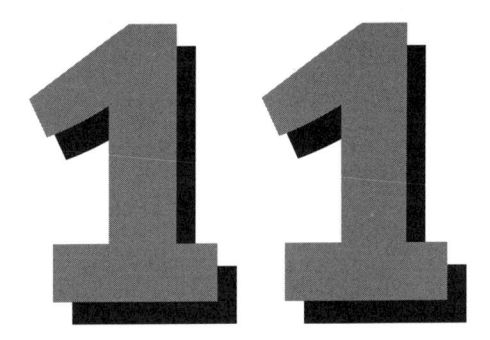

Surveyors will want to see that your hospital's infection control program reduces the risk of infection in patients, employees, and visitors. As they tour your hospital, the surveyors will look for evidence that your infection control program

- effectively monitors and evaluates the potential for infection throughout the hospital;
- is based upon known infection control problems at your institution and in the community, and upon national data on infection trends;
- incorporates infection prevention strategies such as educational classes for staff and closely monitors high risk areas such as the ICU;
- considers the potential risk to everyone in your hospital, such as your patients, employees, and visitors.

Keep these points in mind as you review all of your infection control policies and procedures and gauge your compliance with the infection control standards.

Checklist 11: Infection Control (IC)

Standard	Assessment Point	Yes	No	Example of Compliance	Notes
★ IC.1	Do you have a well-defined, organized, and coordinated IC program that reduces the risk and spread of infection in patients and employees?	☐	☐	The hospital screens laboratory cultures and sensitivity data to identify resistant organisms; the hospital holds annual inservices on proper hand washing techniques; the hospital makes gloves and other personal protective equipment available to all staff.	
★ IC.1 IC.2	Is the hospital's IC program based upon • the hospital's location, size, and patient population? • important epidemiological issues? • local and state health department requirements? • identified infection patterns or trends in hospital, community, or national data? • past infection control problems in the hospital? • current infection control literature and other national sources?	☐ ☐ ☐ ☐ ☐ ☐	☐ ☐ ☐ ☐ ☐ ☐	The hospital has an IC plan, policy, or procedure that describes the hospital's approach to IC; its IC plan is based on data and literature from the Centers for Disease Control and Prevention and IC journals; tuberculosis (TB) prevention is a priority for the hospital because of a community trend showing a rise in the number of identified TB cases.	
IC.1.1	Is the individual who manages your IC program qualified to do so by • certification? • education? • training? • experience?	☐☐☐☐	☐☐☐☐	Your IC manager's current C.V. and training and continuing education documentation indicate that he or she is qualified.	
IC.3	Does the hospital have a well defined system for reporting important IC issues • internally? • externally?	☐ ☐	☐ ☐	The hospital uses logs and reports to update state and local health departments, medical staff, and administration on IC issues.	

The JCAHO Mock Survey Made Simple, 1999 Edition

Checklist 11: Infection Control (IC)

Standard	Assessment Point	Yes	No	Example of Compliance	Notes
🏃 IC.4 IC.5	Does the hospital's IC program • outline strategies to reduce the risk of exposure to or the spread of nosocomial infections? • address potential risks to patients, visitors, and employees? • define methods to manage and control infection outbreaks?	☐ ☐ ☐	☐ ☐ ☐	Policies describe how staff should use personal protective equipment; the hospital has instituted negative air flow handling systems in isolation rooms; a report describes what actions were taken to control an outbreak of chicken pox.	
🏃 IC.6	Does the hospital collect and analyze IC data and use this information to make improvements to the IC program?	☐	☐	Data is collected by tracking and trending infection rates by location, procedure, and diagnosis; performance improvement reports demonstrate that IC data is analyzed and used to develop improvement plans.	
IC.6	Is the hospital's IC program integrated with • the employee health program? • the hospital's performance improvement (PI) program?	☐ ☐	☐ ☐	Preventative vaccines, such as those for hepatitis B and measles, are distributed through the employee health program. PI projects focus on IC issues; reports to PI committees comment on the progress of infection control PI teams.	
IC.6.1	Does the IC program have administrative support?	☐	☐	IC committee meeting minutes document administrative support of the program, such as administrative representation on the IC committee; the IC plan and IC policies/procedures have administrative sign off; the IC department reports its activities to a medical staff quality committee or to the medical executive committee.	

The JCAHO Mock Survey Made Simple, 1999 Edition

Checklist 11: Infection Control (IC)

Standard	Assessment Point	Yes	No	Example of Compliance	Notes
✥ IC.6.2	Does the hospital reduce the risks of infection transmission between patients and staff?	☐	☐	Documents indicate that the hospital has changed to a needleless system; personal protective devices are available to employees who request or need them.	

The JCAHO Mock Survey Made Simple, 1999 Edition

Governance (GO)

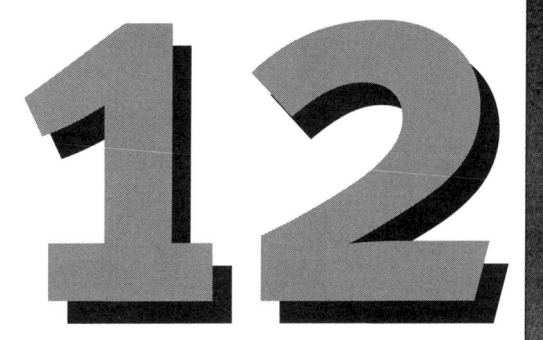

12

Your governing board establishes the tone and culture of your organization, and over the years, it has grown in importance in the eyes of the JCAHO and the community. The governing board has the ultimate responsibility for ensuring that the hospital provides its patients with safe, effective, efficient, and appropriate care.

If your governing board has trouble meeting any of the JCAHO's requirements, it will most likely be in the areas of medical staff participation (GO.2.2) and compliance with legal and regulatory requirements (GO.2.4). Remember that the JCAHO expects a medical staff representative to not only be a member of the board, but to also regularly attend board meetings. In addition, JCAHO surveyors will want to see that the governing board oversees the hospital's compliance with all applicable local, state, and federal requirements.

Checklist 12: Governance (GO)

Standard	Assessment Point	Yes	No	Example of Compliance	Notes
✦ GO.1 GO.2.1	Has the governing board documented or defined in its bylaws • the lines of authority in the hospital? • its role, including who is responsible for planning, management, and operations? • the criteria for board membership? • how it will evaluate its own performance? • the board's legal responsibilities to patients? • whether it must report to an oversight board? • how it should establish a medical staff? • what constitutes a conflict of interest?	☐ ☐ ☐ ☐ ☐ ☐ ☐ ☐	☐ ☐ ☐ ☐ ☐ ☐ ☐ ☐	An organizational chart defines the board's structure and its relationship to hospital administration and medical staff; bylaws describe the governing board's reporting structure, responsibilities and relationship to the hospital—e.g. executive management staff report to the CEO, the CEO and the medical staff report to the board of directors, and the board of directors reports to the corporate or system board.	
✦ GO.2 GO.2.1	Does the governing board oversee and have the ultimate responsibility for • the quality of patient care? • medical staff credentialing? • performance improvement and risk management activities? • budget and finance decisions? • management, planning, and policy decisions?	☐ ☐ ☐ ☐ ☐	☐ ☐ ☐ ☐ ☐	Bylaws define the board's responsibilities; selected board members belong to committees and report on issues, such as professional relations or performance improvement, to the full board; the governing board signs off on various hospital-wide documents, such as the risk management plan, the performance improvement plan, and the hospital budget.	
✦ GO.2.2 GO.2.2.1	Does a medical staff representative attend board of directors meetings?	☐	☐	Governing board bylaws state that the medical staff is represented at board meetings; governing board membership lists include a medical staff representative as an active, voting member of the board; governing board minutes show that the medical staff is represented at board meetings and involved in board level decision making.	

Checklist 12: Governance (GO)

Standard	Assessment Point	Yes	No	Example of Compliance	Notes
✦ GO.2.2 GO.2.2.1	Does the medical staff recommend to the board how best to • organize and structure the medical staff? • appoint and reappoint medical staff members? • terminate medical staff members? • manage due process for medical staff members?	☐☐☐☐	☐☐☐☐	The medical executive committee makes formal recommendations to the board of directors regarding which physicians should be appointed or reappointed.	
GO.2.2.2	Does a medical staff member have the right to apply for board of director membership?	☐	☐	This application process and rationale is outlined in medical staff bylaws, rules and regulations; board membership lists indicate that medical staff members have applied and been accepted to the hospital board.	
GO.2.3	Does the governing board select qualified CEOs based on a candidate's educational background and experience?	☐	☐	The CEO's CV demonstrates that the governing board selected a qualified individual.	
GO.2.4 GO.2.5 GO.2.6	Does the governing board oversee • compliance with all legal and regulatory requirements?	☐	☐	The governing board has assigned various people in the organization to oversee compliance and report on key issues.	
	• the development of key hospital policies and procedures, such as significant medical staff and nursing policy decisions?	☐	☐	The medical staff has developed policies on signing verbal orders, resuscitation, and "No CPR"; the nursing staff has developed a policy allowing nurse extenders to change dressings on wounds.	
	• conflict resolution among leaders?	☐	☐	Governing body bylaws describe the appeals process for addressing medical staff credentialing issues or other grievances.	

The JCAHO Mock Survey Made Simple, 1999 Edition

Management (MA)

13

It's rare for hospitals to fail to comply with the management standards, since most chief executive officers (CEOs) are well qualified and clearly understand their responsibilities. Nevertheless, you should not take this chapter lightly. Surveyors will expect to find evidence that the CEO's management structure and style positively impacts your organization. For example, if the hospital has recently established a new management structure and new lines of responsibility, the survey team will want to see that managers and staff both understand and benefit from these new reporting relationships.

Checklist 13: Management (MA)

Standard	Assessment Point	Yes	No	Example of Compliance	Notes
MA.1	Was the CEO appointed by the governing body?	☐	☐	Governing body minutes document the appointment and reappointment/evaluation process.	
MA.1	Does your CEO manage and effectively operate				
	• your organization, including its physical and financial resources?	☐	☐	Your organizational chart is appropriate for the size and scope of your organization; there is evidence of quality outcomes, budget compliance, strong customer service satisfaction ratings, a capital plan, growing market shares, and a high-caliber medical staff; the CEO has developed a strategic plan to replace outdated facilities and add needed services and bring in new income.	
	• all information and support systems?	☐	☐	Management satisfaction surveys, physician satisfaction surveys, and reports from managed care providers indicate that your information and support systems are satisfactory and a plan for future information and support systems exists.	
	• staff recruitment and retention programs?	☐	☐	Evidence of low turnover rates, strong employee recognition programs, and a competitive wage and employee benefits program.	
MA 1.1	Does your CEO have the appropriate education and experience needed to manage your hospital's services?	☐	☐	A resume or CV on file demonstrates the CEO's qualifications.	

The JCAHO Mock Survey Made Simple, 1999 Edition

Checklist 13: Management (MA)

Standard	Assessment Point	Yes	No	Example of Compliance	Notes
MA.2 MA.2.1	Has your CEO clearly defined who must oversee the hospital's regulatory compliance and respond to the findings of all appropriate regulatory agencies?	☐	☐	Job descriptions clearly identify who is responsible for maintaining compliance with each agency's standards (e.g., the manager of employee health oversees OSHA compliance, the quality resources department oversees JCAHO and Medicare compliance); documented evidence that the manager of quality resources responds to JCAHO Type I recommendations within a specified time frame.	
MA.3	Have the CEO and hospital leaders outlined the lines of responsibility within the hospital?	☐	☐	The CEO and senior leaders worked together to develop the hospital's organizational chart and plan of care.	
MA.4	Does your CEO safeguard human, physical, financial, and information resources in your hospital?	☐	☐	The hospital's CEO and senior leaders have established staff recruitment and retention, safety, capital expenditures, budget, collection, and information integrity policies.	

Medical Staff (MS)   14

Over the years, the medical staff has been forced to become more and more involved in hospital-wide activities. Payors, regulators, and consumer groups have placed increasing pressure on individual practitioners, medical staff leaders, and the hospital to develop new systems and processes that are efficient and effective. To meet these requests, the medical staff and the hospital must work together to improve the quality of the hospital's care, and the hospital must ensure that its medical staff is competent and qualified.

Often, the medical staff has trouble with JCAHO requirements such as:

- documenting its involvement in hospital-wide performance improvement activities;
- developing medical staff bylaws that are consistent with the practices of the medical staff and meet regulatory requirements; and
- maintaining complete, accurate, and up-to-date credentials files.

Keep these issues in mind as you gauge your hospital's compliance with the medical staff (MS) standards. Also, use **Checklist 17: Credentialing** and **Checklist 26: Medical Staff Leaders' Responsibilities** to help you ensure that you meet all of the JCAHO's medical staff requirements.

Checklist 14: Medical Staff (MS)

Standard	Assessment Point	Yes	No	Example of Compliance	Notes
✽ MS.1 MS.1.1 MS.1.1.1 MS.1.1.2 MS.1.1.3	Is your medical staff(s)*: • self-governed? • responsible for the quality of its services? • accountable to the governing board? • comprised of licensed physicians? • required to follow its own policies? • subject to peer review? *Note: Your organization may have more than one medical staff only if it provides care to separate patient populations at geographically distinct sites.	☐☐☐☐☐☐	☐☐☐☐☐☐	The medical staff's bylaws address each of these issues. An organization has merged with another hospital that is located in a town 70 miles away. Each medical staff is separate and distinct, and the patient populations do not overlap.	
✽ MS.2– MS.2.3.6.1 MS.2.5 MS.3.1.1 MS.4.2 MS.5 MS.5.3.2 MS.5.5– MS.5.7 MS.5.8– MS.5.8.2 MS.5.10.1.1 MS.5.10.2– MS.5.10.3 MS.5.14.4 cont'd	Do the medical staff's bylaws, rules, regulations, and/or policies and procedures • define the existence, size, responsibilities, and composition of the medical executive committee (MEC)? • outline requirements for fair hearings, appellate reviews, and automatic and summary suspensions? • describe how the medical staff should be organized?	☐ ☐ ☐	☐ ☐ ☐	The MEC is composed of the chiefs of each medical department, an "at-large" member from each medical staff department, four medical staff officers, the vice president for medical affairs, the hospital's chief executive officer, and the vice president of nursing. The process for fair hearings requires the president of the medical staff to select four impartial medical staff members to serve on the hearing board. The medical staff is organized into five departments—medicine, surgery, pathology, emergency medicine, and radiology; it consists of three categories of membership—active, courtesy, and provisional; it has four officers—treasurer, secretary, president,	

The JCAHO Mock Survey Made Simple, 1999 Edition

Checklist 14: Medical Staff (MS)

Standard	Assessment Point	Yes	No	Example of Compliance	Notes
MS.5.17 MS.6.2– MS.6.5.2 cont'd	• clearly define			and vice president, each of whom are elected for two-year terms.	
	- how to select medical staff officers? - what qualifications these officers should have?	☐ ☐	☐ ☐	Every two years there is a general election to select new officers for a two-year term; a physician must be an active member of the medical staff and in good standing to be an officer; an	
	- when and how an officer may be removed? - how often medical staff meetings must be held?	☐ ☐	☐ ☐	officer may only be removed by an action of the MEC; medical staff departmental meetings are held quarterly and at least 50% of the medical	
	- which method the medical staff will use to communicate with the governing board?	☐	☐	staff must attend; the medical staff communicates with the board of directors through the president of the medical staff.	
	• define how the attending medical staff must supervise residents in teaching institutions?	☐	☐		
	• outline medical staff department directors' responsibilities?	☐	☐	The bylaws state that medical staff department chiefs are responsible for overseeing the clinical and administrative functions of their departments.	
	• describe appointment, reappointment, credentialing, and recredentialing processes and requirements?	☐	☐		
	• note that each medical staff member is responsible for providing their patients with quality care?	☐	☐	The bylaws state that physicians must sign a statement accepting responsibility for the care of their patients when they are appointed.	

Checklist 14: Medical Staff (MS)

Standard	Assessment Point	Yes	No	Example of Compliance	Notes
cont'd	• describe the process for granting temporary privileges?	☐	☐	Bylaws state that temporary privileges can be granted for a period of 30 days, pending primary source verification of license, education, training, and competence.	
	• define how privileges will be reviewed if your hospital doesn't have separate clinical departments?	☐	☐	A sub-committee of the MEC reviews all medical staff members' appointment, reappointment, credentialing, and recredentialing requests and presents its recommendations to the MEC.	
	• require all practitioners to function within the limits of their clinical privileges?	☐	☐	Bylaws state that a physician may only perform those procedures for which he or she has been granted privileges.	
	Were these bylaws developed by the medical staff and approved by the governing board?	☐	☐	Meeting minutes indicate that both the medical staff and governing board sign off on all bylaws.	
MS.2.3.7 MS.2.4 MS.2.4.2	Do medical staff leaders frequently review medical staff bylaws, revise them as needed, and share the revisions with the medical staff?	☐	☐	Medical staff leaders review the bylaws at least every two years; new members of the medical staff must sign statements indicating that they have read the bylaws.	
MS.2.3.8	Do you involve the medical staff in issues that directly impact on its role and responsibility?	☐	☐	Medical staff representatives attend board-level and administrative meetings, such as those of the hospital planning committee, the hospital ethics committee, and the capital equipment task force.	
	Do you have mechanisms in place to ensure medical staff involvement in issues that impact its responsibility?	☐	☐		

The JCAHO Mock Survey Made Simple, 1999 Edition

107

Checklist 14: Medical Staff (MS)

Standard	Assessment Point	Yes	No	Example of Compliance	Notes
MS.2.4.1	Are there any conflicts between the medical staff bylaws and the governing board bylaws?	☐	☐	A conflict might occur if the medical staff bylaws state that a department chief must be board certified but the governing board bylaws state that a department chief may be appointed if he or she is board eligible.	

✦ MS.3– MS.3.1.7, MS.5.1	Does the MEC
	• act on behalf of the entire medical staff?
	• make recommendations to the governing board on
	  - the medical staff's organization and structure?
	  - appointments and reappointments?
	  - clinical privileging?
	  - medical staff participation in performance improvement?
	  - how to remove a physician from the medical staff and hold a fair hearing?
	• follow up on recommendations from clinical departments, divisions, or committees?
		☐☐
		☐
		☐☐☐
		☐☐
		☐
		☐
			☐☐
			☐
			☐☐☐
			☐☐
			☐
			☐
				The MEC recommends to the board of directors which new physicians should be appointed to the medical staff; these recommendations are documented in the minutes of MEC and board of directors meetings; the board of directors acts on these recommendations and sends its responses back to the MEC.	

✦ MS.4– MS.4.2.1.6	Is there a director for each clinical department who is
	• board certified or appropriately experienced in his or her specialty?
	• properly credentialed?
	• responsible for his or her department's
	  - clinical and administrative activities?
	  - performance evaluations?
	  - recommendations for clinical privileging?
		☐
		☐
		☐☐☐
			☐
			☐
			☐☐☐
				The chief of medicine is board certified in internal medicine and has 20 years of experience in internal medicine; this individual reviews departmental budgets, manages all clinical and administrative activities, and makes recommendations to the MEC regarding privileges.	

Checklist 14: Medical Staff (MS)

Standard	Assessment Point	Yes	No	Example of Compliance	Notes
🏃 MS.5.1.1 MS.5.1.2 MS.5.3– MS.5.3.3	Are the hospital's medical staff appointment, re-appointment, credentialing, and recredentialing procedures				
	• approved and implemented by the governing board and the medical staff?	☐	☐	Governing board meeting minutes document their approval.	
	• explained to each new applicant to the medical staff?	☐	☐	A description of the appointment and reappointment process is given to each applicant.	
	• the same for both medical staff members and individual practitioners?	☐	☐	Medical staff chiefs are reappointed according to the same process as all other physicians.	
🏃 MS.5.2 MS.5.4.4.1	Do you have an appeals process and hold fair hearings for medical staff members who				
	• are not granted initial appointment and privileges?	☐	☐	A physician who was not granted privileges may request a hearing, as outlined in the appeals process; hospital and medical staff select the members of the hearing committee.	
	• have their privileges modified?	☐☐	☐☐		
	• have their privileges revoked or not renewed?	☐☐	☐☐		
MS.5.4– MS.5.4.3 MS.5.4.3.1 MS.5.4.3.1.1	Do you have criteria that describe how you: • select new medical staff members? • grant clinical privileges? Are the criteria: • uniformly applied?	☐	☐	Criteria state that all physicians must be board certified or board eligible in their specialties in order to be appointed to the medical staff. The medical staff office does not process applications from any physician who is neither board certified nor board eligible.	

The JCAHO Mock Survey Made Simple, 1999 Edition

109

Checklist 14: Medical Staff (MS)

Standard	Assessment Point	Yes	No	Example of Compliance	Notes
cont'd	• department specific?	☐	☐	All emergency department physicians must be ACLS certified.	
⚑ MS.5.4– MS.5.4.3 MS.5.4.3.1 MS.5.4.3.1.1	For new applicants to the medical staff, do you verify with primary sources their: • licensure? • training and experience? • competence? • ability to perform requested privileges?	☐☐☐☐	☐☐☐☐	Medical staff office personnel send a written request to the applicant's medical school, along with a signed release from the applicant, requesting verification that the applicant attended and completed medical school.	
MS.5.9	Are your appointment and privileging processes non-discriminatory?	☐	☐	A physician is denied privileges in thoracic surgery because he or she does not have sufficient experience and competence, and not because of his or her race, gender, religion, or disabilities.	
MS.5.10– MS.5.10.1.1	During the appointment and privileging process, do you obtain each medical staff applicant's written consent to obtain and review relevant documentation and records?	☐	☐	As part of the appointment application, physicians are asked to sign releases allowing the hospital to verify their education, malpractice history, training, and competence.	
⚑ MS.5.11	Are appointments and clinical privileges granted for a maximum of two years?	☐	☐	A review of applicants' files indicates that the hospital reviews medical staff appointments and clinical privileges every two years.	
⚑ MS.5.12– MS.5.12.3	Do medical staff department chiefs appraise the performance of physicians in their departments before making any reappointment or reprivileging decisions?	☐	☐	Medical staff department chiefs review their staff's compliance with medical record completion and staff meeting attendance requirements.	

The JCAHO Mock Survey Made Simple, 1999 Edition

Checklist 14: Medical Staff (MS)

Standard	Assessment Point	Yes	No	Example of Compliance	Notes
MS.5.13	Does your department chairperson, or chief of service, approve all recommendations for reappointment and reprivileging? Do these recommendations include a review of the individual's: • performance? • health status? • competency? • ability to perform new or expanded privileges?	☐ ☐ ☐ ☐ ☐	☐ ☐ ☐ ☐ ☐	The quality improvement department provides department chiefs with data and information on any problems that were identified during the physician peer review process.	
✪ MS.5.14– MS.5.14.2	Do you delineate clinical privileges to all independently licensed practitioners (LIPs)?	☐	☐	Independently practicing psychiatric nurses and/or social workers must have delineated privileges within the department of psychiatry which specify what activities they may perform; medical staff office personnel provide the operating room, the cath lab, and the endoscopy suite with a list of which physicians are privileged to perform which procedures.	
MS.5.14– MS.5.14.2	Do you ensure that all practitioners, physicians, and LIPs perform only the procedures they are privileged for?	☐	☐	Medical staff office personnel provide the operating room with a list of privileged physicians.	
MS.5.14.3	Do you define the criteria and scope of privileges for contracted physicians?	☐	☐	The radiology department ensures that all contracted physicians are appropriately privileged.	
MS. 5.14.4	Do you have a process for granting temporary clinical privileges which includes at least the following:				

The JCAHO Mock Survey Made Simple, 1999 Edition

Checklist 14: Medical Staff (MS)

STANDARD	ASSESSMENT POINT	YES	NO	EXAMPLE OF COMPLIANCE	NOTES
cont'd	• establishing a time frame for temporary privileges?	☐	☐		
	• conducting primary source verifications of credentials, such as current licensure (phone calls are permitted)?	☐	☐		
	• verifying current competence?	☐	☐		
	• obtaining a recommendation from the applicant's department chair or the president of the medical staff?	☐	☐		
	• obtaining a sign-off by the CEO or designee?	☐	☐		
MS.5.15 MS.5.15.1 MS.5.15.1.1 MS.5.15.1.2 MS.5.15.1.3 MS.5.15.2 MS.5.15.3	When granting privileges, do you consider: • experience and training? • outcomes of care? • results of performance improvement and peer review activity? • specialty board certification?	☐☐☐ ☐	☐☐☐ ☐	At the time of reappointment, the department chief reviews the results of hospital-wide quality and performance activity, risk management and peer review results, and any updates to education and training before he/she decides to reappointment a practitioner to the medical staff. **or** The department chief receives information from the various hospital committees, the QI department, the risk management department, and the medical records department that he/she keeps in the practitioner's department file for review prior to reappointment.	
MS.5.15.4	When privileges are grouped into categories, do you include for each category: • a definition of the range of services provided?	☐	☐	Your organization lists all laparoscopic procedures in its laparoscopic surgery category.	

The JCAHO Mock Survey Made Simple, 1999 Edition

Checklist 14: Medical Staff (MS)

Standard	Assessment Point	Yes	No	Example of Compliance	Notes
cont'd	• standards that applicants must meet to be granted the full category of privileges?	☐	☐	To be awarded privileges for laparoscopic surgery, the practitioner must have completed an approved course, performed a defined number of procedures, and have been observed and found to be competent by the chief or his or her designee on a number of cases.	
MS.5.15.5 – MS.5.15.5.1	Do you coordinate re-appointment and reprivileging decisions with all departments to which a physician is assigned?	☐	☐	The OB/GYN department and the department of medicine work together to make reappointment and reprivileging decisions for a family practice physician who handles patients in each department.	
MS.5.15.6	Do medical staff members understand that they must follow departmental rules and regulations and the authority of their department chairs?	☐	☐	Each medical staff applicant signs a statement noting that he or she will comply with departmental policies and procedures.	
MS.6– MS.6.1	Are physicians' admitting privileges compliant with • state laws? • the hospital's medical staff standards?	☐☐ ☐☐	☐☐ ☐☐	According to state law and medical staff standards, physicians are licensed in the state in which they apply for privileges; each physician must carry one million dollars worth of malpractice insurance.	
MS.6.6– MS.6.7	If you offer psychiatric and/or substance abuse treatment programs, do you • determine when a multidisciplinary treatment plan is appropriate? • require physicians to approve this plan?	☐ ☐	☐ ☐		

The JCAHO Mock Survey Made Simple, 1999 Edition

Checklist 14: Medical Staff (MS)

Standard	Assessment Point	Yes	No	Example of Compliance	Notes
cont'd	If your facility doesn't offer psychiatric and substance abuse treatment programs, do you develop a written plan of care that • defines the treatment plan for the psychiatric or substance abuse problem? • outlines how the physician will implement the treatment plan? • specifies when referrals to or consultations with outside sources are appropriate?	☐ ☐ ☐	☐ ☐ ☐	A multidisciplinary care team develops a care plan to manage a patient who is hospitalized for surgery and has a substance abuse problem; the hospital has a policy that states that because the hospital does not offer psychiatric and substance abuse treatment, patients needing such services are provided with the appropriate consultation, stabilized, and transferred.	
✈ MS.6.8	Do you ensure that patients receive consistently high-quality care throughout the hospital?	☐	☐	Orthopedic surgeons and podiatrists must meet the same privileging criteria to operate on feet.	
MS.7–MS.7.2.1	Do you offer physicians the opportunity to participate in hospital-sponsored continuing medical education programs?	☐	☐	The hospital offers an annual risk management program for all members of the medical staff and provides each member who attends with continuing medical education credits.	
✈ MS.8–MS.8.2.3	Do you involve the medical staff in performance improvement (PI) activities, particularly those affecting the quality of • patient assessment and treatment? • medication use and blood use? • operative procedures? • patient outcomes? • patient and family education? • care coordination throughout the hospital? • medical records completion?	☐☐☐☐☐☐	☐☐☐☐☐☐	The quality improvement department screens all procedures using the SIMS criteria; exceptions to the criteria are referred to the clinical chiefs for review and action as necessary; composite results of all PI activities are reported to the MEC.	

The JCAHO Mock Survey Made Simple, 1999 Edition

114

Checklist 14: Medical Staff (MS)

Standard	Assessment Point	Yes	No	Example of Compliance	Notes
MS.8.3– MS.8.4	Does the medical staff report and appropriately act upon the results of its PI activities?	☐	☐	The chief reviews the results of peer review and PI activities; when a pattern or trend is noted, the chief reviews all of the physician's cases before discussing the problem with the physician.	
	When the findings of PI activities indicate that there may be a problem with the performance of an individual practitioner, do you review 100% of his or her cases?	☐	☐		
❂ MS.8.5– MS.8.5.3	Have you established criteria that help to determine when an autopsy is needed and how to notify the patient's attending physician?	☐	☐	The house officer, or attending physician, obtains the family member's signature and consent before an autopsy can be performed.	

Nursing (NR)

15

Like the standards in the management chapter, the nursing standards are not frequently associated with compliance problems. Occasionally surveyors have been known to question a nurse executive's educational background if she or he has not been exposed to particular specialty areas within your scope of services, but even this should not be a major concern. If the nurse executive is supported by other nursing leaders who serve as knowledgeable experts for the specialties in question, compliance will be easily demonstrated.

Checklist 15: Nursing (NR)

Standard	Assessment Point	Yes	No	Example of Compliance	Notes
NR.1	Does your nurse executive have • a current license for your state? • appropriate education and experience?	☐☐	☐☐	A resume or CV on file demonstrates that the nurse executive is qualified for the position.	
NR.1 NR.2	Does the nurse executive direct all nursing services? Or, if your nurse executive does not directly supervise the nursing staff in all areas, has he or she developed policies and procedures that require nurses to deliver one standard of care to all patients?	☐	☐	The nurse executive chairs a committee that reviews and approves all nursing policies, procedures, standards, and practices.	
NR.3	Does the nurse executive set nursing standards, policies, and procedures?	☐	☐	Meeting minutes document that the nurse executive reviews and signs all policies and procedures concerning nursing practice.	
NR.4	Do nursing leaders oversee and encourage organization-wide performance improvement (PI) activities?	☐	☐	Meeting minutes indicate that the nurse executive participates in and attends governing body, medical executive, and executive/management committee meetings; the nurse executive and nurse leaders participate in cross divisional/departmental PI activities as documented in team rosters and meeting minutes.	

Note: If nurse executive responsibilities are shared, such as in a decentralized model, one person is appointed or elected to be the voice for nursing in decision-making forums for one year or more. A rotation of this responsibility is acceptable.

The JCAHO Mock Survey Made Simple, 1999 Edition

Staff Competency 16

Competency assessments are the biggest source of Type I recommendations for human resources departments. One way to find out how well you are doing is to do a thorough check of your personnel files to make sure you have all of the JCAHO's required personnel and competency information.

To review your records, select a sample of 20 to 25 personnel files from:

- day, evening and night shifts;
- weekend staff;
- full- and part-time staff;
- managers and senior leaders;
- nursing; and
- a variety of other clinical and non-clinical staff excluding your medical staff.

Match these files against the information in the following checklist.

Checklist 16: Staff Competency

Standard	Assessment Point	Yes	No	Example of Compliance	Notes
❇ HR.1	Is there a valid, current job description?	☐	☐	The job description should be applicable to the employee's current duties; it should have been revised and updated at least once in the last three years.	
HR.2	Is there evidence that the individual in question is qualified to do his or her job? Does he or she have the proper • education? • experience? • training?	☐ ☐ ☐ ☐	☐ ☐ ☐ ☐	 The job description should require a certain level of education—e.g. a staff accountant should have a degree in accounting. The job description should specify the amount of experience a person must have—e.g. a supervisor in materials management must have two years of experience in materials management. The job description should specify which employees need additional training—e.g. a nurse in the Coronary Care Unit may be required to have Advanced Cardiac Life Support training.	
❇ HR.2	Has the employee's current license, registration and/or certification been verified?	☐	☐	Current RN/LPN licenses are on file for all of your nursing staff.	
❇ HR.4	When hired, did the employee receive • general hospital orientation?* • department specific orientation?*	☐	☐	There is evidence in the personnel files that employees received general hospital and department-specific orientation.	

The JCAHO Mock Survey Made Simple, 1999 Edition

Checklist 16: Staff Competency

STANDARD	ASSESSMENT POINT	YES	NO	EXAMPLE OF COMPLIANCE	NOTES
HR.4.2	Has the employee received job training, when necessary?	☐	☐	The hospital offers nurses in the critical care unit special training in EKGs.	
✈ HR.4.2	Has the employee received annual education on safety issues such as • general safety management, such as who to call in an emergency or how to protect oneself? • fire/life safety? • safe use of equipment, as applicable? • security? • utilities failures, such as how to handle a power outage, a water main break or a computer system failure? • safe handling of hazardous materials? • emergency preparedness or disaster training?	☐ ☐☐☐☐ ☐☐	☐ ☐☐☐☐ ☐☐	The employee's file indicates that he or she attended annual employee education sessions.	
IM.4	Is there evidence that employees who collect, analyze and/or use data have received appropriate information management training?	☐	☐	Employees who work with the computer system have been trained to use its applications; department managers are trained to use data, as appropriate.	
HR.3.1 HR.4.2	Has the employee received continuing education and annual retraining?	☐	☐	The employee's file indicates that he or she has attended annual inservices related to his or her job, such as annual fire/safety training.	
✈ HR.3.1 HR.4.2 HR.5	Has the employee received an annual criteria-based performance assessment or appraisal?	☐	☐	On the employee's date of hire anniversary, his or her manager conducts an annual performance appraisal, and includes a copy of the appraisal in the personnel files.	

The JCAHO Mock Survey Made Simple, 1999 Edition

124

Checklist 16: Staff Competency

Standard	Assessment Point	Yes	No	Example of Compliance	Notes
❊ HR.3.1 HR.4.2 HR.5	Is there evidence of annual reassessment of appropriate competencies, when applicable?	☐	☐	Each year the department manager reassesses each employee's competency, and includes a copy of the appraisal in the personnel files.	
For non-physicians with patient contact only:					
❊ HR.3.1 HR.4.2	Is there evidence that the employee has received an annual age-specific competency assessment that identifies which • human development knowledge or skills the employee must have? • age-specific patient needs the employee is required to understand and meet?	☐ ☐ ☐	☐ ☐ ☐	Emergency department staff are trained and tested in their ability to recognize both the needs of the children coming into the emergency department and the normal developmental stages of children.	
❊ HR.3.1	During orientation, did you determine which age groups the employee is competent to work with by reviewing the employee's educational background, training and prior experience?* ** applies to employees hired on or after January 1, 1993*	☐	☐	All new hires receive an initial competency assessment that evaluates what training an employee may need before he or she can work with specific patient groups, such as the elderly.	

The JCAHO Mock Survey Made Simple, 1999 Edition

Credentialing 17

Credentialing is critical to your hospital. Your patients trust you to ensure that your medical staff is qualified and competent and provides top quality care. This is precisely why your credentials files are so important—they are proof that the hospital verifies the qualifications of its practitioners.

The credentialing process can be very cumbersome and time consuming, considering the amount of detail and follow-up required to verify a physician's application. Still, these steps are necessary. It is important to remember that you should follow your state's credentialing laws and regulations as well as the JCAHO's requirements. In case of a conflict, follow the stricter standard.

Use this checklist to help you assess the quality of your credentials files. Select a sample of at least 10 to 30 medical staff members from your roster (depending on the size of your organization), and be sure to include both newly appointed staff members, re-appointed staff, and clinical chiefs in your sample. Pull the credentials files for each of these individuals and match them against the requirements listed in the following checklist.

Checklist 17: Credentialing

Standard	Assessment Point	Yes	No	Example of Compliance	Notes
✈ MS.1.1.1 MS.5.4.3	Is there a current copy of the individual's license on file?	☐	☐	A current copy of the individual's license is filed in his or her credential file.	
✈ MS.1.1.1 MS.5.5.1	Is there a current copy of the physician's drug enforcement agency (DEA) registration on file?	☐	☐	A current copy of the physician's DEA registration is filed in his or her credential file.	
✈ MS.1.1.2	Does the individual have delineated clinical privileges?	☐	☐	A physician in the department of surgery has delineated privileges for laparoscopic and general surgery procedures.	
✈ MS.3.1.6.1 MS.3.1.6.1.1	Is there a copy of the individual's appointment or reappointment request that was • recommended by the chief of the department?	☐	☐	A written statement signed by the medical staff chief recommends the individual to be appointed or reappointed to the medical staff.	
	• recommended by the medical executive committee (MEC)?	☐	☐	A copy of the MEC meeting minutes indicates that the individual's appointment or reappointment was recommended to board of directors; a formal recommendation, such as memorandum from the MEC, notes who is recommended for appointment or reappointment.	
	• approved by the board of directors?	☐	☐	A copy of the board of directors' minutes notes that the individual's request for appointment or reappointment was approved.	

The JCAHO Mock Survey Made Simple, 1999 Edition

Checklist 17: Credentialing

Standard	Assessment Point	Yes	No	Example of Compliance	Notes
MS.4.1.1	If the individual is a medical staff chief who was appointed or reappointed after January 1, 1992, is he or she specialty board certified or comparably experienced?	☐	☐	If your chief is not board certified but has effectively led the department for a number of years, the credentials committee can identify and list the experiences that makes him or her qualified to lead the department.	
✈ MS.5.4.3.1	Have you verified with an original source the individual's • license? • education? • training? • references? • competence?	☐☐☐☐☐	☐☐☐☐☐	Documentation proves that you sent formal, written requests to the individual's licensing board, medical school, residency program, and former places of employment to verify the individual's claims.	
MS.5.5.1 MS.5.5.2 MS.5.5.3	Has the individual disclosed all • voluntary or involuntary changes to his or her licensure? • any changes in medical staff membership at any other institution? • any pending malpractice suits or finalized settlements?	☐ ☐ ☐	☐ ☐ ☐	The hospital requests information from the National Practitioners Data Bank, the American Medical Association Physician Masterfile, and the Federation of State Medical Board's Physician Disciplinary Data Bank to help verify the physician's information.	
✈ MS.5.5.3	Is there a current copy of the individual's malpractice insurance policy, indicating that he or she has the appropriate amount of coverage specified in your bylaws?	☐	☐	A current copy of the individual's insurance policy is filed in his or her credential file.	

The JCAHO Mock Survey Made Simple, 1999 Edition

Checklist 17: Credentialing

Standard	Assessment Point	Yes	No	Example of Compliance	Notes
MS.5.7	Does the file contain recommendations from peers regarding the individual's • current competency? • health status? • ability to fulfill medical staff responsibilities?	☐☐☐	☐☐☐	Written letters from peers address each of these areas.	
MS.5.10 MS.5.10.1	Is there a copy of the individual's signed consent to allow hospital administration to obtain information to verify his or her credentials?	☐	☐	The individual's consent to release information must be current, signed, and dated.	
MS.5.10– MS.5.10.3 MS.5.11 MS.5.16	Is there a signed statement from the individual stating that he or she • accepts his or her medical staff responsibilities? • will provide continuous care to patients? • has received copies of the medical staff's by-laws, rules, regulations, policies, and procedures?	☐☐☐	☐☐☐	Such a statement is signed at the time of the individual's initial appointment.	
☙ MS.5.11	Was the individual reappointed to the medical staff within the last two years?	☐	☐	The hospital has a system for tracking all reappointments and ensuring that they occur within the required time frame.	
MS.5.12– MS.5.12.3	Is there evidence that reappointment decisions are based on compliance with medical staff rules and regulations?	☐	☐	Department chiefs base reappointment decisions on physicians' medical record completion rates, compliance with continuing medical education requirements, and level of attendance at medical staff meetings.	

The JCAHO Mock Survey Made Simple, 1999 Edition

Checklist 17: Credentialing

Standard	Assessment Point	Yes	No	Example of Compliance	Notes
🏃 MS.5.12–MS.5.12.3 MS.8.3 MS.8.4	Is there evidence in the file that the decision to reappoint an individual was based on • the results of peer reviews? • the individual's level of participation in performance improvement (PI) activities?	☐ ☐	☐ ☐	The department chief bases his or her reappointment decisions on the results of blood usage, operative and invasive procedures, utilization, and drug usage reviews, and the physician's role in PI activities.	
🏃 MS.5.13	Is there a recommendation from the chief of the department regarding the individual's • performance? • health status? • current competence? • ability to perform expanded privileges, if requested?	☐ ☐ ☐ ☐	☐ ☐ ☐ ☐	Before recommending a physician for reappointment, the chief reviews the physician's number of admissions, the types of patients he or she has treated, the number of reported performance problems, as well as the physician's current health status.	
MS.5.15.5	Has the individual been appointed to at least one medical staff department?	☐	☐	The physician requested and was granted privileges to the departments of medicine and family practice.	

Medical Records 18

Your medical records will help to prove to surveyors that you provide patients with excellent care. During the medical record interview, your surveyors will review a sample of about 20 of your medical records to ensure that they meet JCAHO requirements. Long before their visit, you should review a random sampling of your records to ensure that they are all in good shape.

Use the following checklist to help you gauge whether your medical records are in line with JCAHO standards, or if they need some work. Take approximately 50 to 100 completed medical records, drawn from a cross-section of physicians and services, and compare them to the requirements listed on this form. This will help you determine the most prevalent problems in your documentation, and determine where you should focus your improvement efforts.

Checklist 18: Medical Records

STANDARD	Record: 1	2	3	4	5	6	7	8	9	10
Patient Rights (RI)										
RI.1, RI.1.2.3, RI.1.3.4—There is evidence of a resolved ethical or treatment issue.										
RI.1.1—The patient is admitted and/or transferred based on his or her need for services.										
RI.1.2—The patient and, when appropriate, the family are involved in the patient's care.										
🏃 RI.1.2.1–RI.3—Informed consent is obtained for treatments, procedures, or research participants (benefits, risks, and alternatives are discussed).										
RI.1.2.2—If appropriate, surrogate decision-makers are identified.										
🏃 RI.1.2.4—The patient is asked if he or she has an advance directive, and if so, the advance directive is in the record, or the intent of the advance directive is documented.										
RI.1.2.5–RI.1.2.6—DNR and withholding or withdrawing life-sustaining treatment orders follow hospital policy.										
🏃 RI.1.2.7—The patient and family members' needs are individually addressed during the end of life.										

Note patient record numbers

✓ -met   ✗ -failed   ( ) -comments   N/A -not applicable

The JCAHO Mock Survey Made Simple, 1999 Edition

135

Checklist 18: Medical Records

Note patient record numbers

STANDARD	Record: 1	2	3	4	5	6	7	8	9	10
RI.1.3.4—Patient and/or family complaints are addressed.										
RI.1.3.5—Requested pastoral counseling is provided.										
RI.1.3.6—Individual (non-English-speaking, visually or hearing impaired) patient communication needs are considered.										
RI.2—The procurement and donation of organs and other tissues follow organizational policy.										
Assessment of Patients (PE)										
🏃 PE.1—There is a physical, psychological, and social status assessment.										
PE.1.1—The scope and intensity of further assessments are based on diagnosis, the care setting, desire for care, and response to any previous treatment.										
🏃 PE.1.2—Nutritional status is assessed when indicated by the patient's needs.										
PE.1.3–PE.1.3.1—Functional status is assessed when indicated by the patient's needs (a must for patients referred for rehab services).										

✓-met   ✗-failed   ( )-comments   N/A-not applicable

The JCAHO Mock Survey Made Simple, 1999 Edition

Checklist 18: Medical Records

Note patient record numbers

STANDARD	Record: 1	2	3	4	5	6	7	8	9	10
PE.1.4—Appropriate diagnostic tests are performed to determine any patient needs.										
PE.1.4.1—Records show requests for diagnostic tests provide adequate clinical information.										
PE.1.5—The need for a discharge planning assessment is determined.										
PE.1.6—The initial assessment is completed within the time set by hospital policy.										
PE.1.6.1—The H&P, nursing assessment, and other assessments are completed and in record within 24 hours of admission for inpatients.										
PE.1.7—There is an H&P, indicated diagnostic tests, and a pre-operative diagnosis on the record before surgery is performed (with the exception of emergencies).										
PE.1.7.1—Pre-anesthesia assessment for patients for whom anesthesia is planned.										
PE.1.7.2—If anesthesia is planned, a licensed independent practitioner with appropriate clinical privileges determines the patient is an appropriate candidate.										

✓ -met   **x** -failed   ( ) -comments   N/A -not applicable

The JCAHO Mock Survey Made Simple, 1999 Edition

Checklist 18: Medical Records

Note patient record numbers

STANDARD	1	2	3	4	5	6	7	8	9	10
Record:										
PE.1.7.3—If anesthesia is administered, the patient is reevaluated immediately prior to anesthesia induction.										
PE.1.7.4—The patient's status is assessed on admission to and discharge from the post-anesthesia recovery area.										
PE.1.9.1—Laboratory and pathology services and results are provided on a timely basis through the hospital's laboratories or an approved reference laboratory.										
PE.1.14.2—If patient is getting blood glucose monitored on unit, the results are traceable to the machine used for testing.										
PE.2—The patient is reassessed according to hospital policy.										
🏃 PE.2.2—Reassessment occurs at regular intervals and determines the patient's response to care, according to policy.										
🏃 PE.2.3–2.4—Patient is reassessed when there is a significant change in the patient's condition or diagnosis.										
PE.3—Patient needs are identified and prioritized.										
PE.3.1—Care decisions are based on identified patient needs and priorities.										

✓ -met   x -failed   ( ) -comments   N/A -not applicable

The JCAHO Mock Survey Made Simple, 1999 Edition

Checklist 18: Medical Records

STANDARD	Record: 1	2	3	4	5	6	7	8	9	10
PE.4.2—For patients that need emergency care, assessments and treatment are determined by a LIP.										
PE.4.3—In areas where nursing care is provided, an RN assesses the patient's nursing care needs.										
🏃 PE.5—Infants, children, or adolescent patients are individually assessed for psychosocial needs, development aspects, immunizations, family, or guardian expectations and involvement for treatment.										
🏃 PE.6—Emotionally or behaviorally disordered patients are individually assessed for their history of mental, emotional, behavioral, and substance abuse problems, a mental status examination, problem behaviors, and a psychosocial assessment.										
🏃 PE.7—Substance abuse patients are individually assessed for history of alcohol or drug use, physical problems associated with abuse, family history of substance abuse, spiritual orientation, previous treatment, response to previous treatment, history of physical or sexual abuse, sexual history and orientation.										
PE.8—Patients of suspected abuse or neglect are identified, appropriate consents are obtained, and legally required notifications are issued.										

Note patient record numbers

✓ -met   x -failed   ( ) -comments   N/A -not applicable

The JCAHO Mock Survey Made Simple, 1999 Edition

Checklist 18: Medical Records

Note patient record numbers

STANDARD	1	2	3	4	5	6	7	8	9	10
Record:										

Treatment of Patients (TX)

TX.1—Records show that the care, treatment, and rehabilitation plans are appropriate and individualized.

TX.1.1—Services and settings are identified and used to meet care goals.

TX.1.1.1—There is justification for a patient need that is not addressed.

TX.1.2—Processes of interdisciplinary and collaborative care planning and delivery are used throughout the organization.

TX.1.3—The patient's progress is periodically evaluated against his or her goals and the plan of care.

TX.2.1—If anesthesia is administered, there is a care plan for anesthesia.

TX.2.2—If anesthesia is administered, the anesthesia options and risks are discussed with the patient and/or family.

TX.2.3—There is measurement and assessment of the physiological status during surgery.

TX.2.4.1—Patients are discharged from post-anesthesia care unit by a LIP or by using discharge criteria.

✓ -met   ✗ -failed   ( ) -comments   N/A -not applicable

The JCAHO Mock Survey Made Simple, 1999 Edition

Checklist 18: Medical Records

Note patient record numbers

STANDARD	Record: 1	2	3	4	5	6	7	8	9	10
TX.3.9—The effectiveness of medications for the patient is continually monitored.										
TX.4—Nutrition therapy is planned.										
TX.4.1—For patients at nutritional risk, there is an interdisciplinary nutrition plan that is developed and periodically updated.										
TX.4.2—Authorized individuals prescribe or order nutrition.										
TX.4.5—The response to nutrition care is monitored.										
TX.4.6—Special diet needs and/or altered diet schedules are accommodated.										
🏃 TX.5.1.1–5.1.5—Patients undergoing operative and/or invasive procedures have the following documented - review of patient's history, - review of patient's physical status, - review of diagnostic data, - assessment of risks and benefits, and - assessment of need to administer blood or components.										
🏃 TX.5.2.1–5.2.2—Operative patients have been informed about alternative options, the need for and risk of blood transfusions.										

✓ -met   ✗ -failed   ( ) -comments   N/A -not applicable

The JCAHO Mock Survey Made Simple, 1999 Edition

141

Checklist 18: Medical Records

Note patient record numbers

STANDARD	Record: 1	2	3	4	5	6	7	8	9	10
✈ TX.5.3 — Plans of care for the operative patient are documented before the procedure and should include - a nursing plan; - a plan for the operative or other procedure; - a plan for postprocedure care; - assessment of need for additional diagnostic data; - initial assessment of patient acuity to determine post-procedure care, and - an initial assessment of patient's physical, mental, and neurological status and needs.										
TX.5.4 — Patient's post-procedure period is monitored, including - physiological and mental status; - pathological findings; - IV fluids, drugs, and blood and components; - any unusual events or complications and their management, and - impairments and functional status.										
TX.6.1 — Based on the assessment of the physical, cognitive, behavioral, communicative, emotional, pharmacological, and social needs, a treatment plan for rehabilitation patients includes at least - patient goals for rehabilitation; - rehabilitation goals that address living, learning, and working; - measures with time frames for goal achievement, and - description of facilitating factors as well as barriers to reaching goals.										

✓ -met   ✗ -failed   ( ) -comments   N/A -not applicable

The JCAHO Mock Survey Made Simple, 1999 Edition

Checklist 18: Medical Records

Note patient record numbers

STANDARD	Record: 1	2	3	4	5	6	7	8	9	10
TX.6.2—For rehabilitation patients, qualified professionals implement the rehabilitation plan with the patient and/or family, which include - interventions to reach reasonable goals; - coordinated rehabilitation interventions; - the patient's choices, response to interventions, changes in condition, and progress toward goals, and - advocate support services to create new social support or environmental modifications.										
TX.6.3—Rehabilitation interventions improve or maintain the patient's optimal level of functioning and quality of life.										
TX.6.4—Patient is determined to end rehab services based on written discharge criteria.										
TX.7.1—Patients placed in restraint and/or seclusion have exhausted all reasonable alternatives and have adequate justification and documentation for its use, time-limited orders for each use, and documentation that patients received attention to their needs.										
TX.7.2—Patients given electroconvulsive or other convulsive therapy have adequate justification and documentation for its use, per hospital policy and procedures. Medical records of child and adolescent patients who underwent such therapy must contain the reports of two qualified child										

✓ -met   x -failed   ( ) -comments   N/A -not applicable

The JCAHO Mock Survey Made Simple, 1999 Edition

Checklist 18: Medical Records

STANDARD	\multicolumn{10}{c}{Note patient record numbers}
Record:	1	2	3	4	5	6	7	8	9	10
psychiatrists not directly involved in the patient's care, who have examined the patient, consulted with attending psychiatrist, and documented concurrence with the decision.										
TX.7.3—Patients who had psychosurgery or other surgery for intervention of patient's mental, emotional, or behavioral disorder have adequate justification and documentation for their use.										
TX.7.4—Behavioral modification procedures and aversive conditioning have followed the hospital's policies and procedures.										
TX.7.4.1—Qualified staff review, evaluate, then approve all behavioral management procedures.										
Education (PF)										
PF.1—Learning needs, abilities, preferences, and readiness to learn are assessed.										
PF.1.1—Learning needs assessment considers patient's cultural, religious, emotional, motivational, physical, cognitive, and language status.										

✓-met   x-failed   ( )-comments   N/A-not applicable

The JCAHO Mock Survey Made Simple, 1999 Edition

144

Checklist 18: Medical Records

Note patient record numbers

STANDARD	Record: 1	2	3	4	5	6	7	8	9	10
PF.1.2—Based on age and length of stay of patient, academic needs are assessed and education provided if necessary.										
🏃 PF.1.3—Patient is educated on the safe use of medication.										
🏃 PF.1.4—Patient is educated on the use of medical equipment.										
🏃 PF.1.5—Patient is educated about potential food/drug interactions, nutrition, and modified diets.										
PF.1.6—Patient is educated about rehab techniques to help him or her function more independently.										
PF.1.7—Patient is educated about additional community resources.										
PF.1.8—Patient is educated about how to obtain additional treatment, if needed.										
PF.1.9—Patient and family have been educated and are clear what their responsibilities are for the ongoing health care needs of the patient.										
PF.2—The patient education is interactive.										
🏃 PF.3—Discharge instructions given to the patient and/or family are also given to the organization or individual responsible for ongoing care.										

✓ -met   ✗ -failed   ( ) -comments   N/A -not applicable

The JCAHO Mock Survey Made Simple, 1999 Edition

Checklist 18: Medical Records

Note patient record numbers

STANDARD	Record: 1	2	3	4	5	6	7	8	9	10
PF.4.2—Patient and family education is interdisciplinary.										
Continuum of Care (CC)										
CC.2—The entry process for the patient to a particular service reflects consideration of the appropriateness of the care, including setting and service, individualized needs, and the organization's ability to meet the needs.										
CC.2.1—Criteria define patient information necessary to determine the appropriate care setting or services.										
CC.3—The patient and family are informed about the proposed care during the entry process.										
CC.4—There is continuity of care throughout assessment, diagnosis, planning, and treatment.										
CC.5—There is coordination of care among practitioners and services.										
CC.6–CC.6.1—The patient, if referred or transferred, meets the organization's criteria for referral and transfer. Also, records of emergency patients transferred to other organizations include the reason for transfer, stability of the patient, acceptance by the receiving organization, responsibility during transfer, and follow-up planning if required.										

✓-met   ✗-failed   ( )-comments   N/A-not applicable

Checklist 18: Medical Records

STANDARD	Record: 1	2	3	4	5	6	7	8	9	10
CC.7—Complete discharge summary is exchanged when patients are admitted, referred, transferred, and discharged.										
Leadership (LD)										
🏃 LD.1.6—Patients with same health problems and care needs get the same quality of care throughout hospital (conscious sedation, nursing care).										
LD.1.7-1.7.1—Records confirm the organization follows its approved policies and procedures on the scope of services and care provided by each department.										
Management of Information (IM)										
IM.7.2—Records must contain these items - name, address, date of birth, and legal representative; - legal status if mental health patient; - emergency care given prior to arrival, if any; - conclusions or impressions from H&P; - diagnosis or diagnostic impression; - reasons for admission or treatment; - diagnostic and therapeutic orders, if any; - diagnostic and therapeutic procedures and tests and their results; - operative and other invasive procedures performed, using acceptable terms, including etiology;										

Note patient record numbers

✓ -met   **x** -failed   ( ) -comments   N/A -not applicable

The JCAHO Mock Survey Made Simple, 1999 Edition

Checklist 18: Medical Records

Note patient record numbers

STANDARD	Record: 1	2	3	4	5	6	7	8	9	10
- progress notes by the medical staff and other authorized individuals; - reassessments, if needed; - clinical observations; - response to care; - consultation reports; - every medication ordered or prescribed; - every dose administered and any adverse reactions; - every medication dispensed to inpatient at discharge or to ambulatory patient; - all relevant diagnoses established during care; - any referrals/communication to other providers; - discharge instructions to patients and family; and - discharge summary containing reason for hospitalization, significant findings, procedures performed, treatment given, condition on discharge, and any instructions given to patient or family.										
IM.7.2—A final progress note may be substituted for a summary only for patients with minor problems and less than 48-hour stay, or for newborn infants or normal deliveries. Transfer summary may be used instead of discharge summary only when patients are transferred to different level of hospitalization or residential care within the organization.										
IM.7.3.1—Surgery records show pre-operative diagnosis by LIP.										

✓-met   x-failed   ( )-comments   N/A-not applicable

Checklist 18: Medical Records

STANDARD	Record: 1	2	3	4	5	6	7	8	9	10
IM.7.3.2—Operative report, completed immediately after surgery, describes findings, procedure used, specimen removed, post-operative diagnosis, and name of primary surgeon and any assistants.										
IM.7.3.2.1—Operative report is authenticated and dated by surgeon.										
🏃 IM.7.3.2.2—If the operative report is not filed in medical record immediately after surgery, a progress note is entered immediately.										
IM.7.3.4—Post-operative documentation indicates discharge from PACU by LIP or according to discharge criteria.										
🏃 IM.7.4–IM.7.4.1—For continuing ambulatory care patients, there is a summary list of known significant diagnoses, and conditions, procedures, drug allergies, and medications.										
IM.7.5—Records of emergency visits contain time and means of arrival.										
IM.7.5.1—Records of emergency visits contain a note if patient leaves against medical advice.										
IM.7.5.2—Records of emergency visits contain conclusions at end of treatment, including final disposition, condition, and instructions for follow-up.										

Note patient record numbers

✓ -met   ✗ -failed   ( ) -comments   N/A -not applicable

The JCAHO Mock Survey Made Simple, 1999 Edition

Checklist 18: Medical Records

Note patient record numbers

Standard	1	2	3	4	5	6	7	8	9	10
Record:										
IM.7.5.3—If authorized, a copy of emergency services provided is available to practitioner providing follow-up.										
IM.7.6—Significant clinical information is entered within appropriate time frames.										
🏃 IM.7.7—Staff follow medical staff rules on who is qualified to accept verbal orders and the authentication of orders that carry a potential hazard for a patient within the time frame defined in medical staff rules.										
🏃 IM.7.8—All entries show author, date, and authentication; and all entries made by house staff are countersigned by supervising physicians.										
IM.7.9—All relevant inpatient, ambulatory care, emergency, urgent, or immediate care records are assembled when patient receives care.										
Medical Staff (MS)										
MS.6.1 & 6.2.2—Only individuals privileged to admit patients and perform an H&P do so.										
MS.6.2—If patient is admitted for inpatient treatment, H&P is performed by a physician privileged to do so.										

✓ -met   **x** -failed   ( ) -comments   N/A -not applicable

The JCAHO Mock Survey Made Simple, 1999 Edition

Checklist 18: Medical Records

Note patient record numbers

STANDARD	1	2	3	4	5	6	7	8	9	10
Record:										
MS.6.2.2.1—Records show that when LIPs provide care, physicians confirm their findings prior to major interventions.										
MS.6.2.2.2—For dental patients, dentist performs part of H&P relating to dentistry.										
MS.6.2.2.3—For podiatry patients, podiatrist performs part of H&P relating to podiatry.										
MS.6.3—Staff follow medical staff rules for H&P on outpatients, and medical records reflect compliance.										
MS.6.4—Records show that practitioners who perform surgical or invasive procedures practice within the scope of their delineated privileges.										
MS.6.5—Records show that each patient's general medical condition is the responsibility of a qualified member of the medical staff.										
MS.6.5.2—Consultation by a physician or LIP is obtained under defined circumstances.										

✓ -met   ✗ -failed   ( ) -comments   N/A -not applicable

The JCAHO Mock Survey Made Simple, 1999 Edition

151

Physicians' Offices and Ambulatory Care Sites

19

If your hospital or health care system owns any physician offices or ambulatory care sites, you need to ensure that these facilities comply with the JCAHO's standards. And, while most of the JCAHO's standards are based on common sense and shouldn't present a problem, you do need to take the time to verify that each of these facilities, such as primary care clinics, specialty clinics, cancer centers, rehabilitation services, and physician offices, is in compliance.

Consistency is the watchword here and each physician office and ambulatory care site will probably need to work closely with hospital representatives to bring its practice in line with the hospital's. The public expects to receive the same standard of care throughout your hospital system, and it's up to you to ensure that each physician office or ambulatory care site offers this consistent, high quality care.

Checklist 19: Physicians' Offices and Ambulatory Care Sites

STANDARD	ASSESSMENT POINT	YES	NO	EXAMPLE OF COMPLIANCE	NOTES
RI.1.1	Do you treat all patients with respect?	☐	☐	A policy supports respect for the individual; no patient is treated disrespectfully regardless of circumstances.	
RI.1.1	When you cannot fulfill a patient's request for services, do you refer him or her to another facility for treatment?	☐	☐	Referrals are made to appropriate agencies and providers who are willing and able to provide requested services; the hospital extends its case management services for all high risk cases.	
⚑ RI.1.2 RI.1.2.1.1	Are all patients involved in decisions about their care, including the decision to participate in research protocols or to give their informed consent for a procedure?	☐	☐	The physician's office or ambulatory care site follows the hospital's patient treatment policies; a review of medical records documents good practice and use of informed consent.	
RI.1.2.2	Are patients' families involved in all treatment decisions, as appropriate?	☐	☐	A policy supports family involvement in patient care decisions whenever appropriate, such as when a patient is mentally incompetent.	
⚑ RI.1.3– RI.1.3.6 IM 2–IM.2.2	Do you respect the patient's need for • confidentiality? • privacy?	☐ ☐	☐ ☐	The physician's office or ambulatory care site follows the hospital's patient record confidentiality policies. Gowned waiting areas are away from general traffic; exam rooms do not open up to traffic areas; discussions are conducted out of the earshot of other patients.	

Checklist 19: Physicians' Offices and Ambulatory Care Sites

STANDARD	ASSESSMENT POINT	YES	NO	EXAMPLE OF COMPLIANCE	NOTES
cont'd	• security?	☐	☐	The office's location was selected with patient safety in mind and has adequate security staff; patients' valuables are protected when they undergo procedures and cannot safeguard their belongings.	
	• complaint resolution?	☐	☐	Hospital patient representatives are available to resolve any patient conflicts; training records prove that staff have been taught how to handle patients and family members who voice concerns; staff try to resolve patient problems on their own, and if this does not work, they refer them to patient representatives.	
	• pastoral counseling?	☐	☐	Staff training records demonstrate that staff have been taught how to handle an untoward event and how to access a chaplain or other pastoral service for a patient.	
	• communication?	☐	☐	Interpreters are used for foreign-speaking patients and hearing impaired patients, and special services are offered to blind patients, as appropriate to your population.	
🏃 RI.1.4	Do you inform patients of their rights?	☐	☐	A patient rights statement is posted in every waiting area; in locales where at least 10% of the population is non-English speaking, rights are translated and posted in the predominant language(s).	

Checklist 19: Physicians' Offices and Ambulatory Care Sites

STANDARD	ASSESSMENT POINT	YES	NO	EXAMPLE OF COMPLIANCE	NOTES
RI.4–RI.4.2	Do you comply with the hospital's code of ethics?	☐	☐	Marketing, advertising, and billing practices are in line with the hospital's code of ethics; billing practices are explained to patients; staff are oriented to the hospital's code of ethics.	
🏃 PE.1	Do you perform an age-specific, interdisciplinary assessment of each patient?	☐	☐	A tailored, modified version of the hospital's assessment form is used in all physician offices and ambulatory care sites.	
PE.5	Does this assessment address the patient's physical and mental status?	☐	☐		
	Is it individualized for infants, children, and adolescents?	☐	☐		
PE.1.2	Is a patient's nutritional status assessed when appropriate?	☐	☐	Caregivers screen for nutritionally at-risk patients during all patient assessments; these at-risk patients receive a full nutritional assessment.	
PE.1.4	Do you order diagnostic tests when warranted?	☐	☐	Following assessment, all necessary testing is ordered and arranged through the physician's office or ambulatory care site; all imaging requests are accompanied by relevant clinical data.	
	Is your request for a diagnostic test accompanied by all relevant clinical data?	☐	☐		
PE.1.5	As you conduct assessments, do you try to identify problems in the patient's home which might undermine your treatment plan?	☐	☐	The hospital's case management staff are available to help arrange community services for patients, if needed.	

The JCAHO Mock Survey Made Simple, 1999 Edition

157

Checklist 19: Physicians' Offices and Ambulatory Care Sites

Standard	Assessment Point	Yes	No	Example of Compliance	Notes
PE.1.7	Prior to ambulatory surgery or an ambulatory invasive procedure, do you complete the patient's history and physical, nursing assessment, and any other screening assessments?	☐	☐	A pre-procedure assessment is performed for any patient undergoing an invasive procedure; a short form history and physical, similar to that used by the hospital for an invasive procedure, is completed, along with the equivalent of a nursing assessment.	
PE.1.10– PE.1.14.2	Are laboratory tests performed in compliance with the JCAHO standards and federal and/or state regulations?	☐	☐	All tests are performed by trained personnel according to established protocols and are subject to quality controls.	
PE.3	Do you use the information you gather during assessments to prioritize a patient's care needs?	☐	☐	All care decisions are based on patient assessments; the information from all assessment activities is integrated into the plan of care.	
PE.3	Do you have procedures that define • how you will be notified of abnormal test results? • how you should act on abnormal test results?	☐ ☐	☐ ☐	Abnormal results are communicated promptly to a physician and appropriate follow-up is documented in the patient record.	
PE.4.1	Have you defined what type of assessment each practitioner in the office can perform?	☐	☐	An assessment policy defines the scope of assessment for each professional, including registered nurses; this policy is consistent with practice in other ambulatory areas of the hospital.	
PE.1.8 PE.8	Do you assess all patients to determine if they might be abuse victims?	☐	☐	All staff who conduct patient assessments use a check sheet that prompts them to look for signs of child, sexual, spousal, and elder abuse.	

Checklist 19: Physicians' Offices and Ambulatory Care Sites

Standard	Assessment Point	Yes	No	Example of Compliance	Notes
✈ TX.1 TX.1.2	Do you base your patient care, treatment, and rehabilitation plans on the results of patient assessments?	☐	☐	All protocols can be individualized based on the needs of the patient.	
TX.1.1.1	If you cannot meet a patient's assessed needs, do you document this in the medical record?	☐	☐	If a patient requires services not provided by the physician's office or ambulatory care site, the patient's needs are documented and referrals are made; a patient's refusal to receive needed treatment is documented.	
TX.1.2	Can you demonstrate that care is collaboratively planned and provided by qualified staff?	☐	☐	Medical records prove that physicians discuss patient care plans with registered nurses, nurse practitioners, or other physicians as necessary.	
TX.1.3	Do you review each patient's goals and progress? Are these goals revised when needed?	☐ ☐	☐ ☐	Each patient receiving treatment is assessed by the office team during every visit.	
✈ TX.3	Do you follow all of the hospital's policies and procedures for ordering, dispensing, administering, and monitoring medication?	☐	☐	The hospital's medication use policies and procedures, particularly those regarding the use of samples, extend to the physician's office or ambulatory care site; a nurse from the physician's office belongs to the hospital's pharmacy and therapeutics committee.	
TX.4	Do you ensure that patient's nutritional needs are assessed and met?	☐	☐	Nutritional problems are documented on the summary list, which is reviewed at every visit; patients are interviewed about their food intake; weight and growth measurements are taken.	

Checklist 19: Physicians' Offices and Ambulatory Care Sites

Standard	Assessment Point	Yes	No	Example of Compliance	Notes
PF.1 PF.1.1	Do you teach patients and their families how to address their patients' health care needs?	☐	☐	All patient education efforts are coordinated between all disciplines; the office uses standard educational handouts to teach patients how to handle common health problems; patients are referred to community health education programs and hospital-run support programs for further education, as appropriate.	
PF.4	Do you work with hospital staff to develop interdisciplinary approaches to patient and family education?	☐	☐	The physician office or ambulatory care site works with the hospital to develop educational materials; the hospital's resource center serves as a central repository for educational materials.	
CC.2	Do caregivers determine where a patient should be referred for further treatment?	☐	☐	Caregivers review the criteria defining which patients will be accepted into a specialty service; acutely ill patients are transferred to the emergency room.	
CC.3	Do you routinely explain the proposed plan of care to patients and their families?	☐	☐	Office procedures require caregivers to discuss recommended care plans and goals with patients and their families; this discussion is documented in the medical record.	
CC.4	Do you offer continuously high quality care through the patient's course of treatment?	☐	☐	Each patient is assigned a primary care physician; this physician is responsible for discussing the patient's progress with the patient and his or her family; office staff call patients to remind them of upcoming appointments and offer them written information on preventative care and available community resources.	

The JCAHO Mock Survey Made Simple, 1999 Edition

Checklist 19: Physicians' Offices and Ambulatory Care Sites

Standard	Assessment Point	Yes	No	Example of Compliance	Notes
CC.4	Do you provide patients with after-hours care?	☐	☐	The physician is part of a coverage group; all calls are directed to the covering physician by the answering service; the next morning, physicians receive reports from the covering physician on all after hours calls.	
CC.5	When a patient requires multiple outpatient visits, do you ensure that all caregivers are up-to-date on the patient's progress?	☐	☐	Team meetings are held to ensure that all caregivers are up-to-date on a patient's progress; problem lists for patients with high-risk diagnoses are posted on-line in the health care network's information system.	
🏃 CC.6 CC.6.1	Do you ensure that patients are safely referred or transferred to other providers?	☐	☐	Whenever a patient is referred or transferred to another provider, the name of this provider and the date and time of the patient's first visit with this individual is noted in the patient's record and given directly to the patient and his or her family; case managers in the hospital help transition patients to new providers, if needed.	
CC.7	If you refer a patient to another setting, do you ensure that the next care provider receives all of the patient's clinical information?	☐	☐	A patient care referral form prompts staff to forward pertinent clinical information to new care providers.	
🏃 PI.3–PI.5	Do you measure and assess the quality of your processes and outcomes?	☐	☐	The physician's office measures the completeness of its assessments of elderly patients, the waiting time for initial appointments, and the number of readmissions for patients who have been through its diabetic education program.	

The JCAHO Mock Survey Made Simple, 1999 Edition

Checklist 19: Physicians' Offices and Ambulatory Care Sites

Standard	Assessment Point	Yes	No	Example of Compliance	Notes
LD.1.1–LD.1.1.1	Are your services consistent with the hospital's mission and strategic plans?	☐	☐	The physician office or ambulatory care site follows the hospital's mission to improve the health status of the community by helping clients stay healthy.	
🏃 LD.1.3.3.1	Do you collect data on patient satisfaction?	☐	☐	Surveys are conducted every quarter to gauge patients' satisfaction with the quality of patient care, staff courtesy, security, and patient and family education; the results of these surveys are summarized and trended over time and are shared with staff as part of your performance improvement (PI) program.	
LD.1.7.1	Do you have a written plan of care that defines your goals and scope of services?	☐	☐	Your written plan of care is consistent with the hospital's plan of care and outlines the services you provide and your hours of operation.	
LD.1.8	Do your leaders participate in the hospital's decision-making process?	☐	☐	Your practice manager reports to the Vice President of Managed Care, who is a member of the hospital's management and strategic planning committees.	
🏃 HR.1 HR.2	Do you have job descriptions for all staff, a system to evaluate staff competency, and a staffing plan?	☐	☐	Job descriptions, a competency tool, and a manning table have all been developed and implemented.	
HR.1 HR.2	Do you verify job candidates' qualifications?	☐	☐	A review of personnel records demonstrates that you verify the licenses and other qualifications of all job applicants.	

The JCAHO Mock Survey Made Simple, 1999 Edition

162

Checklist 19: Physicians' Offices and Ambulatory Care Sites

Standard	Assessment Point	Yes	No	Example of Compliance	Notes
HR.2 LD.1.5.2	Do you have a flexible staffing plan that adjusts for peaks and valleys in the community's need for services?	☐	☐	The physician office has three part-time staff members who are cross-trained in front office procedures and exam set-ups, and who are available to work a full-time schedule if needed.	
HR.3.1	Do you encourage staff to pursue educational opportunities on their own?	☐	☐	The physician's office orients all new staff and assigns them to a preceptor; the office budget includes resources for in-house training and attendance at educational seminars as needed.	
HR.4	Do you offer appropriate staff training and orientation in-house?	☐	☐		
🏃 HR.5	Do you evaluate staff competency?	☐	☐	Staff are evaluated at least annually using an age-specific competency tool; the results from these evaluations determine the assignments for all staff members; if an action plan for remediation is required, it is developed jointly with the staff member at the time of the evaluation.	
🏃 IM.2.1 IM.2.2	Do you protect the integrity of all data and information in your organization?	☐	☐	All physician's offices and ambulatory care sites in the hospital network safeguard information by using passwords and required fields and tracking users.	
IM.2.3	Do you ensure that records are protected from loss, destruction, tampering, or unauthorized use?	☐	☐	Paper records are stored in a sprinklered, locked area; only authorized personnel have access to patient records.	
IM.5	Are patient records readily available?	☐	☐	The hospital's system-wide information system includes a core of information on every patient with a medical record; additional information is available through prompt retrieval of the complete medical record.	

The JCAHO Mock Survey Made Simple, 1999 Edition

Checklist 19: Physicians' Offices and Ambulatory Care Sites

Standard	Assessment Point	Yes	No	Example of Compliance	Notes
☸ IM.7.4	Do you maintain a summary list for every patient who is seen on a continuing basis (three visits or more) which describes all • significant medical diagnoses and conditions? • significant operative and invasive procedures? • drug allergies? • medications prescribed for or used by the patient?	☐☐☐☐	☐☐☐☐	The core record on the hospital's information system stores and updates this information at every visit and is accessible by all care providers in the system; a manual summary list is maintained in the record and is used by all care providers who see the patient.	
☸ IM.8	Do you use aggregate data to support managerial decisions, operations, and the PI process?	☐	☐	Aggregated data on patient wait times, canceled appointments, and unauthorized visits to the emergency room is collected and assessed to help make staffing, patient education, and practice protocol decisions.	
☸ IM.8	When you make appointments, do you note in a log or register • the patient's name, age, and gender? • the date and time of the appointment (or date and time of arrival for a walk-in patient)? • the reason for the visit? • whether there is a need for a return visit? • the time of the patient's departure?	☐☐ ☐☐☐	☐☐ ☐☐☐	Your facility is part of the hospital's on-line scheduling system, which collects and maintains this information.	
IM.9	Do staff have access to relevant literature and other information resources?	☐	☐	The hospital's resource center or library serves the entire hospital community; poison control information is on-line to all physician office sites.	
EC.1 EC.1.1	Do you comply with all ADA requirements for handicap accessibility?	☐	☐	The office's entrance, exit, washrooms, and exam rooms are all handicap accessible.	

164

Checklist 19: Physicians' Offices and Ambulatory Care Sites

Standard	Assessment Point	Yes	No	Example of Compliance	Notes
🏃 EC.1.3– EC.1.9 EC.2.2– EC.2.9	Have all staff received orientation and training in the areas of • safety? • security? • the handling of hazardous materials and waste? • emergency preparedness? • life safety? • the safe handling of medical equipment? • using utility systems?	☐ ☐ ☐ ☐ ☐ ☐ ☐	☐ ☐ ☐ ☐ ☐ ☐ ☐	All of these topics are covered in employee orientations and refresher sessions are held annually; periodic safety tours help keep employees knowledgeable; key safety information is posted on staff bulletin boards.	
🏃 EC 2.9 EC.2.10	Do you hold quarterly fire drills? Do you check all fire extinguishers to ensure that they are in working order? Are evacuation routes posted? Are exit signs visible? Are egress and ingress routes clear and free of obstacles?	☐ ☐ ☐ ☐ ☐	☐ ☐ ☐ ☐ ☐	Your facility is included in the hospital's fire safety program and participates in scheduled and unannounced drills and inspections of equipment.	
EC.2.11	Do you have a hazard surveillance program?	☐	☐	Hazard surveillance is conducted every six months; the hospital's standard safety checklist is used and findings are included in the quarterly report to the hospital's safety committee.	

The JCAHO Mock Survey Made Simple, 1999 Edition

165

Checklist 19: Physicians' Offices and Ambulatory Care Sites

Standard	Assessment Point	Yes	No	Example of Compliance	Notes
EC.2.12–EC.2.14	Do you maintain, test, and inspect your • fire detection and extinguishing systems? • medical equipment? • utility systems?	☐ ☐ ☐	☐ ☐ ☐	Your facility receives all equipment and systems maintenance tests required by hospital policy; this is performed by the hospital's biomedical engineering department or is out-sourced to a qualified vendor.	
EC.5	Do you enforce a non-smoking policy?	☐	☐	As a provider of health care services and in keeping with the mission of the hospital, all physician offices and ambulatory care sites have strict no smoking policies.	
IC.3	Do you report all infectious diseases?	☐	☐	Your facility follows a written procedure for reporting infectious diseases; the hospital's infection control staff is available to answer any of the office staff's questions.	
IC.4 IC.5	Do you: • reduce infection risks? • control outbreaks of infection?	☐ ☐	☐ ☐	The physician office recently renovated the waiting area to increase air exchange; two new hall sinks for staff hand washing were installed; the pediatric office has eliminated toys in its waiting area and encourages parents to bring a familiar toy with the child; two staff with chicken pox were given compensatory time off to reduce the risk of infecting patients and other staff.	
MS.6.2.1–MS.6.2.2.3	Do only privileged caregivers perform patient histories and physicals? Are these histories and physicals approved by the medical staff?	☐ ☐	☐ ☐	Nurse practitioners are credentialed through the medical staff prior to being assigned to the physician office or ambulatory care site; credential committee minutes indicate that nurse practitioners are privileged to perform histories and physicals.	

The JCAHO Mock Survey Made Simple, 1999 Edition

Checklist 19: Physicians' Offices and Ambulatory Care Sites

Standard	Assessment Point	Yes	No	Example of Compliance	Notes
MS.2.5	Do you supervise house staff who rotate to the physician office or ambulatory care site?	☐	☐	Physicians who are active members of the physician practice serve as preceptors when residents work in a physician's office or ambulatory care setting; the preceptor must be on-site during office hours and review all new treatments and care plans with residents.	
NR.1 NR.2 NR.3	If you provide nursing services, do these nurses follow and help develop • nursing policies and procedures? • nursing plans of care? Do these nurses participate in the hospital's • decision making process for nursing care? • PI activities?	☐ ☐ ☐ ☐	☐ ☐ ☐ ☐	If your facility is not part of the hospital's patient care services division, it is represented on the nursing standards committee by a nurse practitioner; all of your nursing policies and procedures are approved in that forum; your nurses participate in all hospital-required education sessions, such as those designed to explain a new drug distribution system.	
If you offer rehab services:					
TX.6 TX.6.2	Do you prepare and follow written care plans for each patient?	☐	☐	Rehabilitation plans address the patient's goals, how these goals will be achieved and which factors may influence the outcome; the rehab service documents patients' progress and failures.	
TX.6.3	Can you demonstrate how effective each patient's plan of care is?	☐	☐	Each patient's progress is documented on the plan of care.	

The JCAHO Mock Survey Made Simple, 1999 Edition

Checklist 19: Physicians' Offices and Ambulatory Care Sites

Standard	Assessment Point	Yes	No	Example of Compliance	Notes
TX.6.4	Are discharge criteria used to determine whether a patient is ready to be discharged from a rehabilitation program?	☐	☐	Discharge criteria are set when the plan of care is developed and are modified as needed during treatment; the patient is kept informed of his or her progress.	
PE.1.3.1	Do you perform a complete functional assessment before a patient is referred for rehabilitation? *Note: This would only occur in orthopedic or physiatry offices that have their own rehab departments.*	☐	☐	All new rehabilitation patients are required to have a full functional assessment.	

IV Conscious Sedation vs. Anesthesia

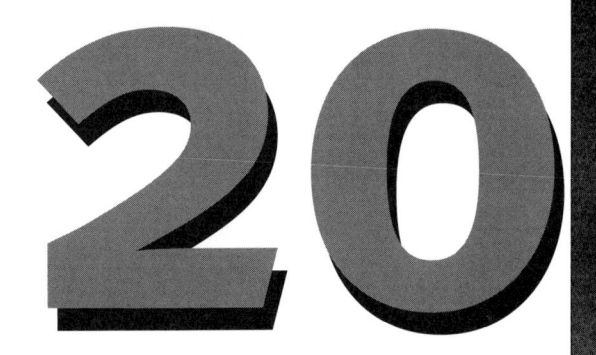

20

Many hospitals have trouble defining exactly what constitutes anesthesia or sedation. Is it a class of drugs, a patient "state," or a location? These questions are at the center of the confusion between anesthesia and sedation.

It is important to recognize that the JCAHO defines anesthesia as the loss of a patient's gag reflex and ability to breathe on his or her own. And, surveyors will want to see that your hospital's definition matches this guideline. You should develop a list defining exactly what does and does not constitute anesthesia in your organization. Be sure to consider each situation, location, or drug which might cause a patient to lose his or her protective reflex, as well as how a patient's size, sensitivity to drugs, and age will impact the results of sedation. Remember, if you believe a patient may lose his or her protective reflex, then the JCAHO's anesthesia standards will apply.

The key to compliance with the JCAHO's anesthesia and sedation requirements is to remember that they do not apply merely to procedures performed in the operative suite. These standards should be followed anywhere that anesthesia or IV conscious sedation is administered, such as outpatient centers, ambulatory clinics, and many other patient care settings.

Checklist 20: IV Conscious Sedation vs. Anesthesia

Standard	Assessment Point	Yes	No	Example of Compliance	Notes
☘ PE.1.7.1 PE.1.7.3 TX.2 TX.2.1	On all patients scheduled to receive anesthesia, do you perform • a pre-anesthesia assessment? • a reassessment immediately prior to surgery?	☐ ☐	☐ ☐	Before a procedure, a member of the anesthesia department evaluates and assesses all patients scheduled to receive anesthesia to ensure that they are appropriate anesthesia candidates.	
☘ PE.1.7.1 PE.1.7.3 TX.2 TX.2.1	Do you document the results of anesthesia assessments in the medical record and use them to develop anesthesia care plans?	☐	☐	An anesthesiologist documents his or her assessment of a patient's readiness and appropriateness for anesthesia in a pre-anesthesia note; anesthesia care plans are communicated to all appropriate caregivers.	
☘ PE.1.7.1 PE.1.7.3 TX.2 TX.2.1	Can you identify all situations in which a patient may lose his or her protective reflex?	☐	☐	The hospital has identified all situations, locations, and medications that may cause a patient to lose his or her protective reflex; the hospital has a policy stating that when the potential exists for the patient to lose his or her protective reflex, the JCAHO's anesthesia standards must apply.	
☘ PE.1.7.2	Before you administer anesthesia, do you ensure that the chosen anesthetic is appropriate?	☐	☐	Caregivers consider a patient's age, physical condition, sensitivities, emotional status, weight, and physical status when selecting an anesthetic.	
☘ PE.1.7.4 TX.2 TX.2.3 TX.2.4 TX.2.4.1	Are anesthesia patients assessed and monitored • before receiving anesthesia? • while anesthesia is being administered? • throughout their stay in the post-anesthesia care unit (PACU)?	☐ ☐ ☐	☐ ☐ ☐	Recovery room nurses assess patients' physical and mental status when they first arrive in and are discharged from the PACU; the anesthesia administration record notes that the anesthesiologist monitors the patient while anesthesia is administered.	

The JCAHO Mock Survey Made Simple, 1999 Edition

Checklist 20: IV Conscious Sedation vs. Anesthesia

Standard	Assessment Point	Yes	No	Example of Compliance	Notes
TX.2 TX.2.1	Do you anesthetize obstetric or emergency department patients within 30 minutes of their documented need for anesthesia?	☐	☐	Medical records indicate that obstetric patients receive requested anesthesia within the set time limit.	
🏃 TX.2.2	Do you explain the potential hazards of anesthesia to the patient and his or her family?	☐	☐	The hospital has a policy requiring informed consent for anesthesia; documentation in medical record indicates that the hospital follows this policy.	
🏃 TX.2.4.1	Do you discharge patients from the PACU only upon the instructions of a qualified practitioner?	☐	☐	Recovery room nurses determine that a patient is ready to be discharged from the PACU based on assessment criteria developed by the medical staff.	
PI.4.5.2	Do you examine all adverse events associated with anesthesia to look for performance improvement opportunities?	☐	☐	The department of anesthesiology reviews aggregated data on anesthesia patients' outcomes to look for improvement opportunities; the chief of anesthesia reviews and evaluates all untoward events following anesthesia and acts on these findings.	
🏃 LD.1.6	Do hospital leaders ensure that every anesthesia patient receives the same quality of care throughout the hospital, no matter where anesthesia is administered?	☐	☐	A policy identifies all situations that qualify as anesthesia and outlines how anesthesia should be administered throughout the hospital, from the general operative suite to the GI lab.	

The JCAHO Mock Survey Made Simple, 1999 Edition

Restraint and Seclusion

21

In July 1996, the JCAHO introduced 25 new restraint and seclusion standards. These standards caused a tremendous amount of confusion and difficulty in most hospitals, and sent many organizations scrambling to revise their entire approach to restraint and seclusion. In November 1998, the JCAHO revised those standards for surveys and the standards went into effect on January 1, 1999. These revisions came as a result of a task force set up by the JCAHO to address the many concerns that hospitals had about the previous standards. Since the restraint standards came out in 1996, they have topped the list for Type 1 recommendations. In fact, two of the JCAHO's top 10 Type I findings in the first six months of 1998 were related to restraints standards.

While the JCAHO has been responsive to the concerns of the hospitals, it has not lost sight of its focus on reducing the use of restraints in acute medical/surgical hospital settings. The newly revised standards help to demystify some of the previously hazy areas, such as what qualifies as restraint and separate out the medical surgical use of restraints from restraint use in a psychiatric setting. (Please note that we have divided the restraints standards into two sections to correspond with the JCAHO's revisions: Standards for Behavioral Health Patients, and Standards for Acute Medical and Surgical Patients. Refer to the *CAMH* to determine which standards you must follow.) In addition, the new standards bring out some marked changes from the previous standards, such as allowing a nurse to initiate restraint in the absence of an LIP as long as the nurse obtains a verbal or written order from an LIP within 12 hours.

To effectively manage restraint and seclusion in your organization and meet the JCAHO's standards, you should determine answers to the following questions:

- Which restraint and seclusion policies and procedures must be in place?
- How will you document your compliance with these policies and procedures?
- Who makes the decision to use restraint and/or seclusion? Are these individuals appropriately qualified?
- How do you work to improve your hospital's performance in the area of restraint and seclusion? Can you prove that you've reduced the amount of inappropriate use of restraint and seclusion?
- Do you have protocols? Have they been appropriately approved?
- Do you have a defined, organization-wide approach to the use of restraints that has been endorsed by your organization's administrative and clinical leadership?

Use the following checklist to help you evaluate your restraint and seclusion program and ensure that it is compliant with the JCAHO's standards.

Checklist 21: Restraint and Seclusion

Standard	Assessment Point	Yes	No	Example of Compliance	Notes
\multicolumn{6}{l}{*Standards for Behavioral Health/Psychiatric Patients*}
\multicolumn{6}{l}{These standards apply to the use of restraint/seclusion in behavioral health and psychiatric settings, including designated psychiatric or behavioral health beds in an acute medical-surgical hospital.}
Policies and Procedures					
🏃 TX.7	Did you develop your restraint policies and procedures with multidisciplinary input and approval from • the medical staff? • administration?	☐ ☐	☐ ☐	The hospital has a policy, developed with input from the medical, nursing, and emergency department staff, defining how restraint and/or seclusion should be used in emergency situations; this policy was approved by the medical executive committee and signed by the CEO.	
🏃 TX.7 TX.7.1 TX.7.1.1.1	Do your policies and procedures: • identify, explain, and define the role each discipline plays in restraint and seclusion?	☐	☐	The hospital's policy on restraint use clearly states that a physician or a licensed independent practitioner (LIP) must initiate the order for restraint and a qualified, trained RN may implement it.	
	• specify when it is appropriate to use restraint and/or seclusion?	☐	☐	Policy defines when it is and isn't appropriate to use restraint and/or seclusion; policy states that it is not appropriate to use restraint for staff convenience.	
	• require caregivers to document and justify the use of restraint and/or seclusion?	☐	☐	Policy requires nurses to observe restrained patients at least every hour and document their findings on a restraint flow sheet.	
	• describe how to use restraint and/or seclusion safely?	☐	☐	The hospital's restraint policy requires qualified, trained individuals to observe restrained patients at least every hour and to document their status;	

Checklist 21: Restraint and Seclusion

Standard	Assessment Point	Yes	No	Example of Compliance	Notes
cont'd	• limit the use of restraint and/or seclusion to situations in which there is clear clinical justification?	☐	☐	policy also specifies that restraint orders may not exceed 24 hours. The hospital has guidelines that clearly state which situations are clinically appropriate for restraint and/or seclusion.	
TX.7.1.3	Do your policies and procedures require staff to base their decision to use restraint and/or seclusion on the results of patient assessments?	☐	☐	You do not base the use of restraints and seclusion on a history of previous use. Instead you assess each patient to determine if, under the current circumstances, there is clinical justification for and no alternative to restraint and/or seclusion.	
TX.7.1.3	Do you have a policy that requires staff to be competent to administer restraint and/or seclusion?	☐	☐	The hospital has developed restraint and seclusion education and training programs for staff; the hospital evaluates the competency of these staff members at least annually.	
TX.7.1.3	Have you defined in a policy how restraint and/or seclusion use should be documented in the medical record?	☐	☐	The hospital has defined what constitutes clinical justification for restraint and seclusion, how patients in restraint and/or seclusion should be reassessed, and how this information should be noted in the medical record.	
TX.7.1.3 TX.7.1.3.1.1 TX.7.1.3.1.3 TX.7.1.3.2.5 TX.7.1.3.2.6	Do you have a policy that requires caregivers to • maintain patients' personal rights and dignity while they are restrained or secluded?	☐	☐	Hospital policy requires restrained patient to be treated respectfully, properly clothed, frequently assessed for food, fluid, and toileting needs, and to have their personal needs met in privacy.	

Checklist 21: Restraint and Seclusion

Standard	Assessment Point	Yes	No	Example of Compliance	Notes

cont'd	• provide a restrained or secluded patient with
	  - a safe, clean environment?
	  - a comfortable room temperature?
	  - personal privacy?
		☐☐☐	☐☐☐	The hospital's seclusion room is appropriately ventilated, clean, and has proper furnishings that pose no threat to patients.	

	• address a patient's emotional and physical needs, such as those for
	  - food?
	  - personal hygiene?
	  - physical exercise?
		☐☐☐	☐☐☐	Caregivers perform passive, ROM exercises with restrained patients.	

	• assess a patient before selecting a particular mode of restraint and/or seclusion?	☐	☐	A patient assessment may reveal that 24 hour supervision can be used in place of restraint and/or seclusion.	
	• use the least restrictive restraint and/or seclusion mode available?	☐	☐	A sitter, 24 hour observation, a quiet controlled setting, or a watchful family member may be alternatives to restraint and/or seclusion.	
	• frequently monitor and reassess restrained or secluded patients?	☐	☐	Hospital policy requires caregivers to monitor restrained or secluded behavioral management patients every fifteen minutes.	
	• discontinue the use of restraint and/or seclusion as soon as possible?	☐	☐	Time limited orders for restraint can only be renewed by a LIP.	
✈ TX.7.1.3.2.7	Do you have a policy or procedure that identifies who is • authorized to give verbal/written orders for restraint and/or seclusion?	☐	☐	The hospital permits LIPs, such as physician's assistants (PAs), psychologists, and nurse practitioners, to write restraint and/or seclusion orders.	

The JCAHO Mock Survey Made Simple, 1999 Edition

Checklist 21: Restraint and Seclusion

STANDARD	ASSESSMENT POINT	YES	NO	EXAMPLE OF COMPLIANCE	NOTES
cont'd	• permitted to implement a verbal order?	☐	☐	The hospital allows only qualified, trained staff, such as RNs who have been appropriately trained, to implement restraint and/or seclusion.	
	• authorized to implement restraint and/or seclusion in an emergency situation?	☐	☐	Trained staff such as RNs or PAs are permitted to implement restraint and/or seclusion in an emergency for a period of one hour.	
	• responsible for renewing or discontinuing restraint and/or seclusion?	☐	☐	A licensed independent practitioner must review all emergency restraint and/or seclusion orders.	
TX.7.1.3.2.7	When a patient is restrained or secluded for behavioral health purposes, you follow a policy that requires you to • notify an LIP within one hour of implementation? • secure the LIP's authorization for continued use?	☐ ☐	☐ ☐	Hospital policy requires an LIP to review restraint and/or seclusion orders for behavioral health patients.	
✦ TX.7.1.3 TX.7.1.3.2.8	Do you have a policy that limits an LIP's time-limited restraint and/or seclusion order to • a maximum of 24 hours per order? • 4 hours for adults, 2 hours for children aged 9–17, and 1 hour for children less than 9 years old in primary behavioral health situations?	☐ ☐	☐ ☐	Patients must be reassessed within the time limit of the original order before restraint and/or seclusion can be renewed for another period—for example, prior to the expiration of a physician's two-hour seclusion order for a child with a primary behavioral disorder, the physician reassessed the patient and determined that the order should be renewed for one more two-hour period.	
TX.7.1.3 TX.7.1.3.2.8	Do you have a policy that allows staff to remove a patient from restraint and/or seclusion before the order expires?	☐	☐	Medical records note that staff who removed a patient from seclusion before the LIP's original order expired reinstituted the seclusion when the	

The JCAHO Mock Survey Made Simple, 1999 Edition

Checklist 21: Restraint and Seclusion

Standard	Assessment Point	Yes	No	Example of Compliance	Notes
cont'd	Do you allow staff to reinitiate an order if the problem behavior recurs during the time frame of the original order?	☐	☐	original behavior recurred during the time frame of the original order.	
✈ TX.7.1.3 TX.7.1.3.2.8	Do you have policies that • require an LIP to assess a patient before a time-limited order is renewed? • define how, where, and when a PRN order may be used?	☐ ☐	☐ ☐	Documentation in the medical record indicates that LIPs reassess patients before time-limited orders are renewed. PRN orders may be used for a patient recovering from anesthesia or who is medicated and on a ventilator.	
TX.7.1.3.1– TX.7.1.3.1.2	Do you use approved, criteria-based clinical protocols to direct restraint use?	☐	☐	The medical staff has approved criteria-based protocols allowing nurses to implement restraint without a written order, such as restraining a patient on a ventilator who receives a medication that may cause agitation or confusion.	
Education and Training					
TX.7.1.1.3	Do you educate staff on the proper use of restraint and/or seclusion?	☐	☐	Staff who apply restraint and/or seclusion must receive special training and pass a competency assessment on an annual basis.	
TX.7.1.1.4	Do you explain to patients and their families why restraint and/or seclusion is used?	☐	☐	Staff spend time with patients and their families explaining how and why restraint and/or seclusion are used.	

The JCAHO Mock Survey Made Simple, 1999 Edition

179

Checklist 21: Restraint and Seclusion

Standard	Assessment Point	Yes	No	Example of Compliance	Notes
✦ TX.7.1.3.1.4	Do you assess the competency of staff who implement restraint and/or seclusion?	☐	☐	Hospital-sponsored inservices maintain staff competency.	
Documentation					
✦ TX.7.1.3.1.1 TX.7.1.3.3	Do you have evidence in your medical record that restraint and/or seclusion • is used for clinically justified reasons? • is based upon an identified need? • is applied and used in a manner that is consistent with hospital policies and procedures? • preserves patients' rights, dignity, and well being? • is implemented by qualified, trained staff? • is overseen by an LIP? • is reassessed at the frequency defined in your policies and procedures?	☐ ☐ ☐ ☐ ☐ ☐ ☐	☐ ☐ ☐ ☐ ☐ ☐ ☐		
Performance Improvement					
TX.7.1.1.5 TX.7.1 TX.7.1.2	Do you improve the quality of your restraint and seclusion policies and procedures by • regularly monitoring restraint and/or seclusion use as part of your performance improvement program? • gathering and evaluating aggregate data on - the use of restraint and/or seclusion in all units and all shifts?	☐ ☐	☐ ☐	Nursing constantly monitors the use of restraint and/or seclusion and reports its finding to the hospital's quality committee.	

The JCAHO Mock Survey Made Simple, 1999 Edition

Checklist 21: Restraint and Seclusion

Standard	Assessment Point	Yes	No	Example of Compliance	Notes
cont'd	- multiple episodes of use on the same patient? - a high use of restraint on a particular unit or area? • developing tools and strategies to reduce and eliminate the use of restraint and/or seclusion? • redesigning patient care processes to reduce or eliminate restraint and/or seclusion use? • developing preventative strategies?	☐ ☐ ☐ ☐ ☐	☐ ☐ ☐ ☐ ☐		
TX.7.1.1.7	Do you look for alternatives to restraint and/or seclusion?	☐	☐	Twenty-four-hour supervision is used in place of restraint and/or seclusion when appropriate, such as when managing elderly, confused, or agitated patients.	

Standards for Acute Medical and Surgical Patients

These standards apply to the use of restraint and seclusion in a typical medical/surgical hospital under non-psychiatric or behavioral health circumstances, such as protective restraint used in a recovering brain injury or stroke patient.

Standard	Assessment Point	Yes	No	Example of Compliance	Notes
TX.7.5	Have you developed organizational policies that • clearly define your organization's position/philosophy on the use of restraint? • are endorsed and supported by the medical staff, nursing, and administrative leadership? • utilize criteria, standards or guidelines to identify and define those situations where restraint may be appropriate? • address : - education and training?	☐ ☐ ☐	☐ ☐ ☐	The hospital's policy on restraint use clearly states that the administration, board, and medical staff support a restraint-free environment. In light of this position, restraint of medical/surgical patients may be used only when all other options and alternatives have been exhausted and the patient continues to pose a threat to him or herself and/or others. The hospital has established staff education guidelines, which and are included in the policy and procedure, along with	

The JCAHO Mock Survey Made Simple, 1999 Edition

Checklist 21: Restraint and Seclusion

Standard	Assessment Point	Yes	No	Example of Compliance	Notes
cont'd	- staffing? - education of patients and families? - alternatives to restraint?	☐☐☐	☐☐☐	criteria to assist staff in determining which alternative methods to employ and when restraint has become the final option.	
TX.7.5.1	Do you monitor and evaluate the use of restraint? Do you utilize these results to reduce the use of restraint and to improve processes, protocols, and documentation?	☐	☐	As part of the hospital's PI plan, restraint use is reviewed to determine that it is appropriately used—that is, that restraints are used in situations where all other methods for protecting the patients have been unsuccessful, and that all standards for monitoring and assessing the patients were followed. The hospital intensely reviews and analyzes any negative patterns or trends, and any untoward events, and takes corrective measures.	
TX. 7.5.2	Do your restraint policies and procedures • provide for the patient's physical and emotional needs? • provide for the patient's safety? • consider the patient's need for privacy and dignity? • explain all alternatives to restraint? • identify risk factors associated with the use of restraint? • address how to help the patient and family to understand the need for restraint? • define the frequency and content of observation, assessment, and reassessment?	☐ ☐☐ ☐☐ ☐ ☐	☐ ☐☐ ☐☐ ☐ ☐	The hospital has several policies and procedures on the use of restraint, including Care of the Patient in Restraint, which addresses nursing care, patient safety measures, assessment procedures, methods to support the patient's psychological health, and alternatives to restraint. A restraint flow sheet was developed to ensure consistency in patient evaluation and documentation. The medical executive committee, the vice president of nursing, and the hospital's chief executive officer approve all restraint policies and procedures.	

Checklist 21: Restraint and Seclusion

Standard	Assessment Point	Yes	No	Example of Compliance	Notes
cont'd	• require time-limited orders for restraint that do not exceed 24 hours before reassessment by the LIP? • outline what must be documented in the record? • specify that each episode of restraint must be documented? • require approval by the medical staff, nursing, and administration?	☐ ☐ ☐ ☐	☐ ☐ ☐ ☐		

TX. 7.5.3,
TX.7.5.3.1
	Does the use of restraint require:
	• the patient to meet and approved protocol?
	or
	• the written order, not to exceed 24 hours, by an LIP?
	or
	• if initiated by a nurse in the absence of an LIP, a written or verbal order within 12 hours after the initiation of restraint?
	and
	• renewals:
	  - to be written by an LIP?
	  - daily after the first 24 hours?
	  - after the patient has been reassessed to determine continued need?
		☐
		
		☐
		
		☐
		
		☐☐☐
			☐
			
			☐
			
			☐
			
			☐☐☐
				Hospital policy states that an LIP must give the order for restraint except when initiated by a nurse following a protocol, or if the nurse is unable to reach the physician and the criteria for restraint use has been met. Renewals for restraint must be written by the patient's attending physician after he or she has assessed the patient's need to continue restraints.
				
				or
				
				Hospital policy permits the nurse who is caring for the patient to initiate restraint without a written physician order, provided that all other methods have been tried and that the attending physician is not available. The nurse must follow up with the attending physician within 12 hours to obtain a written or verbal order. Renewals for restraint must be written by the physician and require a patient assessment to determine whether continued restraint is necessary.	

The JCAHO Mock Survey Made Simple, 1999 Edition

Checklist 21: Restraint and Seclusion

Standard	Assessment Point	Yes	No	Example of Compliance	Notes
TX. 7.5.3.2	Do your restraint protocols include criteria that define and explain: • the diagnoses, procedures, or conditions to which the protocol applies? • who can initiate restraint? • how restraints are to be applied? • what is included in patient monitoring? • assessment and reassessment procedures? • how and when restraint may be terminated? • documentation requirements? Are all protocols approved by the medical staff, nursing, and administration?	☐ ☐☐☐☐☐☐	☐ ☐☐☐☐☐☐	The hospital has a protocol—approved by the medical staff, nursing, and administration—for utilizing restraints on intubated patients to prevent self-extubation, which might compromise the patient's medical condition.	
TX.7.5.4	Do you have a mechanism to ensure that all patients who are restrained are regularly monitored at least every two hours for the following: • proper application of the restraint? • patient safety? • need for continued use of restraint? • skin integrity? • physical and emotional status? • preservation of patient's personal rights and dignity?	☐☐☐☐☐☐	☐☐☐☐☐☐	Nursing has established a protocol for providing care to the patient in restraints. The protocol includes time frames for observation, required observations, and a checklist that must be completed at every observation.	
TX. 7.5.5	Do you have a policy that requires documentation on • each episode of restraint? • why restraint was initiated? • what alternatives were tried? • results of patient assessment and monitoring?	☐☐☐☐	☐☐☐☐	The hospital has developed a documentation flow sheet that requires staff to document each of the elements listed in the question for TX.7.5.5 (at left). Nursing monitors the completion and accuracy of this tool as part of nursing's PI plan.	

The JCAHO Mock Survey Made Simple, 1999 Edition

Checklist 21: Restraint and Seclusion

Standard	Assessment Point	Yes	No	Example of Compliance	Notes
cont'd	• significant changes in patient behavior or condition? • changes to care as a result of restraint? • termination of restraint? • use of protocols when applicable?	☐ ☐☐☐	☐ ☐☐☐		

The JCAHO Mock Survey Made Simple, 1999 Edition

185

Equipment and Utility Preventative Maintenance

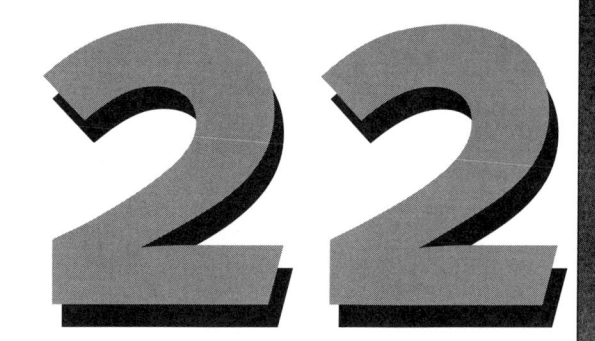

22

The JCAHO requires you to ensure that your hospital is a safe environment for patients, visitors, and staff. This means that you must continually check and care for your equipment and utilities to prevent safety problems.

Because each hospital has a vast amount of equipment that is used by a number of different people with varying skill levels, designing and implementing a continuous preventative maintenance program can be an overwhelming job. The best way to tackle this problem is to review your utilities management, life safety, and equipment management plans to identify what equipment should be included in your preventative maintenance program. You can either include all pieces of medical equipment and utilities systems in your preventative maintenance plan, or you can develop criteria to help you determine which items to include.

Next, review the biomedical engineering office's and the plant operation department's preventative maintenance logs and schedules and compare this documentation to your preventative maintenance list and verify that you meet all of the requirements listed in this checklist.

Checklist 22: Equipment and Utility Preventative Maintenance

Standard	Assessment Point	Yes	No	Example of Compliance	Notes

⚡ EC.1.7 EC.2.12	Do you conduct inspections, testing, and preventative maintenance on
	• fire alarm and fire detection systems quarterly?
	• the automatic fire signal notification system quarterly?
	• automatic fire extinguishing systems, including the following:
	  - fire pumps, under no flow, weekly?
	  - fire pumps, under flow, annually?
	  - water storage water level alarms, semi-annually?
	  - water storage temperature alarms, monthly (during cold weather)?
	  - drains, annually?
	  - fire department connections, quarterly?
	  - kitchen extinguishing devices, semiannually?
	• portable fire extinguishing systems (inspected monthly, given preventative maintenance annually)?
	• all circuits in your fire alarm system including the following:
	  - signal devices, quarterly?
	  - tamper switches and water flow devices, semi-annually?
	  - audible/visible building alarms, annually?
	• all smoke control devices annually?
	• all automatic smoke doors annually?
	• all automatic fan controls annually?
	• all air handling systems annually?
		☐☐ ☐☐☐ ☐ ☐☐☐☐ ☐☐ ☐☐☐☐☐	☐☐ ☐☐☐ ☐ ☐☐☐☐ ☐☐ ☐☐☐☐☐	You've developed and follow an inspection and testing schedule or calendar; you document all safety checks using a computerized schedule or log; the hospital has developed a preventative maintenance schedule which requires staff to perform preventative maintenance on the critical components of the fire alarm system; the hospital maintains careful documentation demonstrating that all checks are performed.	

The JCAHO Mock Survey Made Simple, 1999 Edition

Checklist 22: Equipment and Utility Preventative Maintenance

Standard	Assessment Point	Yes	No	Example of Compliance	Notes
EC.1.8 EC.2.13	Before you purchase or use any new equipment, do you ensure that it meets the criteria defined in your equipment management plan?	☐	☐	Your purchasing department notifies plant operations or biomedical engineering when new equipment is purchased so that the new items can be evaluated before they are put to use.	
🏃 EC.1.8 EC.2.13	Does your equipment management plan describe • the purpose of each piece of equipment? • the risks, hazards, and known problems associated with each piece of equipment? • how frequently each piece of equipment should be inspected?	☐☐ ☐☐ ☐	☐☐ ☐☐ ☐	Your plan states that ventilators and cardiac monitors are high risk equipment that are critical to patient care; the plan also indicates that your preventative maintenance schedule meets manufacturer's requirements and addresses any known problems you've had with the equipment.	
🏃 EC.1.9 EC.2.14	Have you identified and selected which critical utility systems must receive preventative maintenance?	☐	☐	Your preventative maintenance plan requires you to check the safety of electrical circuits, sprinkler heads, and water lines to ensure that your automatic fire extinguishing system is operational.	
🏃 EC.1.9 EC.2.13 EC.2.14	Do you have a current inventory of all of the equipment and critical utilities systems listed in your equipment management plan?	☐	☐	You have an easily updated (e.g. computerized), readily available list of the equipment and critical utility systems that need preventative maintenance.	
🏃 EC.1.9 EC.2.14	Are preventative maintenance schedules based upon a regular 12 month inspection cycle or • the experience of organization? • manufacturers' recommendations? • your safety committee's approval?	☐☐☐	☐☐☐	Your inventory of essential pieces of medical equipment and critical components of your utility systems is the basis for your preventative maintenance schedule; your preventative maintenance schedule is staggered to ensure that the work load is steady but light throughout the year; you maintain documentation proving that you conduct preventative maintenance at regular intervals.	

The JCAHO Mock Survey Made Simple, 1999 Edition

Checklist 22: Equipment and Utility Preventative Maintenance

STANDARD	ASSESSMENT POINT	YES	NO	EXAMPLE OF COMPLIANCE	NOTES
🏃 EC.2.13	Have you set equipment inspection, testing, and preventative maintenance schedules for each piece of equipment in your equipment management plan?	☐	☐	The hospital's preventative maintenance and testing schedules correspond with manufacturer's recommendations.	
EC.2.13	Do you conduct monthly biological testing of • water used in dialysis? • sterilizers?	☐☐	☐☐	Water samples from both your sterilizer and the water you use for dialysis are examined for microorganisms which might cause infection or illness.	
EC.2.13 EC.2.12 EC.2.14	Do you document all inspections, tests, and preventative maintenance performed on all equipment, and note any • problems or opportunities for improvement? • actions taken or recommendations made to resolve issues?	☐☐	☐☐	The hospital documents all preventative maintenance efforts and all equipment inspections and summarizes the information for the safety committee; this information is documented in safety committee reports or action plans.	
	Do you report this information to administration and/or your safety committee?	☐	☐		
🏃 EC.2.14	Do you conduct monthly tests of all emergency generators for • at least 30 minutes? • 30% of the name plate rating or 50% of the greatest known load? • all automatic transfer switches?	☐☐☐	☐☐☐	Tests of emergency generators are conducted once a month to ensure that they perform properly; the results of all tests are documented.	

The JCAHO Mock Survey Made Simple, 1999 Edition

The Seven Environment of Care Plans

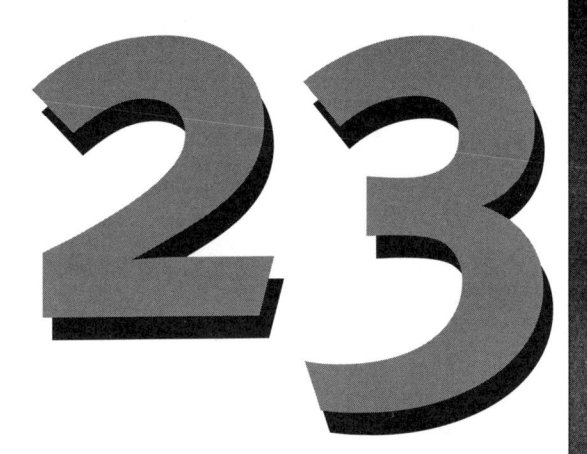

23

The Joint Commission requires hospitals to address the following important environment of care issues:

- safety management;
- security management;
- hazardous materials and wastes;
- emergency preparedness;
- life safety management;
- equipment management; and
- utility management.

It's up to your hospital to decide whether it wants to address these issues in one comprehensive plan or in seven individual plans. All that matters to your surveyors is that you meet each of the requirements listed in this checklist.

Checklist 23: The Seven Environment of Care Plans

Standard	Assessment Point	Yes	No	Example of Compliance	Notes
Safety Management Plan					
⚑ EC.1.3 EC.2.2	Does your safety management plan describe • how to identify, report, and reduce hazards and risks within the hospital and on hospital grounds?	☐	☐	The facilities management department inspects the hospital's grounds and buildings and reports their findings to the safety committee; the biomedical engineering department conducts preventative maintenance checks on all hospital equipment covered by the equipment management plan and reports all findings to the safety committee.	
	• who oversees safety management?	☐	☐	The hospital may designate a safety officer, a safety committee, or a member from administration to oversee safety in the hospital.	
	• how to handle product recalls and alerts?	☐	☐	The hospital has a policy describing who manages all product recalls and how these recalls should be handled.	
	• how to conduct safety inspections?	☐	☐	Safety committee members have developed an inspection checklist and take turns using it to inspect different areas of the hospital; this checklist prompts individuals to look for items like fire doors that don't close properly and blocked doors.	
	• how to report the results of all safety risk assessments?	☐	☐	The results of daily environmental services rounds and weekly administrative rounds are reported to the safety committee and administration.	

The JCAHO Mock Survey Made Simple, 1999 Edition

Checklist 23: The Seven Environment of Care Plans

STANDARD	ASSESSMENT POINT	YES	NO	EXAMPLE OF COMPLIANCE	NOTES
cont'd	• how to handle identified problems?	☐	☐	The hospital has established a reporting process which encourages all employees to report their safety questions to the safety chairperson, who will then present them to the safety committee.	
	• how to monitor at least one performance standard?	☐	☐	The safety officer monitors and reports on the results of annual and semi-annual safety inspections to the safety committee.	
	• when you should review safety policies and procedures?	☐	☐	Each month, the safety committee reviews a different department's safety policies and procedures.	
	• when staff should be trained on safety management?	☐	☐	The hospital's orientation curriculum focuses on hospital-wide, department-specific, and job-related safety issues.	
Security Management Plan					
🏃 EC.1.4 EC.2.3	Does your security management plan describe • how to maintain a safe, secure environment for patients, employees, and visitors?	☐	☐	Employees may report security issues through a security hotline; the security department investigates and reports all security problems.	
	• who is responsible for security management?	☐	☐	The chief security officer oversees the hospital's security program.	
	• who has access to sensitive areas of the hospital?	☐	☐	The hospital identifies which areas are high risk, such as the pharmacy, the operating room, and the nursery; the security management plan identifies who has access to these areas.	

Checklist 23: The Seven Environment of Care Plans

Standard	Assessment Point	Yes	No	Example of Compliance	Notes
cont'd	• how to identify employees, patients, and visitors?	☐	☐	All visitors receive badges when they enter the building, which they must display in a visible location.	
	• how to maintain control of the hospital during a disaster, a civil disturbance, a media event, or a major security threat?	☐	☐	A policy describes what the security force's assigned role is during an emergency, whom it should notify of the disturbance, and when and whom it should call for assistance; in the event of a bomb threat, security officers seal off the area, evacuate patients and employees, and notify local police and any other necessary authorities.	
	• how to handle security problems?	☐	☐	Employees may report security issues via a security hotline; security investigates problems and prepares written reports for the safety committee.	
	• which performance standard should be monitored?	☐	☐	The chief security officer monitors the security force's response to emergency codes and reports on this quarterly to the safety committee.	
	• how staff should be trained on security?	☐	☐	The hospital teaches employees how to minimize a security risk, report a security incident, and handle a security emergency.	

Checklist 23: The Seven Environment of Care Plans

Standard	Assessment Point	Yes	No	Example of Compliance	Notes
Hazardous Materials and Wastes Plan					
EC.1.5 EC.2.4	Does your hazardous materials and waste plan describe how to				
	• safely manage hazardous materials and wastes?	☐	☐	The hospital has a list of approved chemicals that may be purchased and used; there is a policy defining where chemicals can be stored, who can handle them, and what protective equipment must be used; there is a policy describing how to dispose of hazardous wastes, such as placing infectious wastes in red bagged containers.	
	• conduct quality control activities to ensure that all hazardous materials are handled safely?	☐	☐	Employees are monitored to ensure that they wear and use appropriate protective equipment.	
	• document and manage hazardous material spills, exposures, or accidents?	☐	☐	The hospital has an established plan for managing any kind of exposure; employees know whom to call, such as the lab or facilities staff, to respond to an incident; the outcomes of all hazardous spills, exposures, or accidents are reported to the safety committee; safety procedures are located in each department's safety manual; department managers review these procedures with staff at least once a year.	
	• inventory of all hazardous materials and wastes?	☐	☐	Each department has established a list of chemicals used in their area; all lists are kept in a central location and updated annually.	

The JCAHO Mock Survey Made Simple, 1999 Edition

Checklist 23: The Seven Environment of Care Plans

STANDARD	ASSESSMENT POINT	YES	NO	EXAMPLE OF COMPLIANCE	NOTES
cont'd	• teach employees how to manage hazardous materials and wastes as applicable to their jobs?	☐	☐	Staff are taught how to safely handle hazardous materials and waste, how to avoid health risks associated with exposure to a hazardous waste in hospital orientations and in-services.	
	• monitor at least one performance standard for the management of hazardous wastes and materials?	☐	☐	The laboratory department manager monitors how well the chemical spill team responds to emergencies and reports on this quarterly to the safety committee.	

Emergency Preparedness Plan

🏃 EC.1.6 EC.2.5	Does your emergency preparedness plan describe • how the organization should respond to disasters and other emergencies?	☐	☐	Employees are taught to dial an emergency number and have a hospital telephone operator announce "Dr. Disaster" over the PA system in an emergency.	
	• how to initiate the disaster plan and notify staff that it has been initiated?	☐	☐		
	• each department's role in a disaster?	☐	☐	Each department should have specific procedures describing how staff should respond to a disaster.	
	• who oversees and coordinates the hospital's response to a disaster?	☐	☐	An administrator on call may be designated to coordinate and oversee the hospital's response to a disaster, such as making sure that all alternative care sites are operational, that triage is functioning properly, and that supplies have been delivered.	

The JCAHO Mock Survey Made Simple, 1999 Edition

Checklist 23: The Seven Environment of Care Plans

Standard	Assessment Point	Yes	No	Example of Compliance	Notes
cont'd	• how to provide adequate staff coverage during a disaster?	☐	☐	Each department manager establishes a disaster staffing plan for his or her department; this may include bringing in on-call staff, utilizing agency staff, or pulling staff from non-patient care areas.	
	• where you will provide emergency care?	☐	☐	Your plan defines overflow areas and alternative care locations throughout the hospital—for example, in an emergency, the outpatient physical therapy area could be used to treat minor wounds.	
	• how to handle triage?	☐	☐	The hospital plans to flow patients through the emergency department to a house officer and a nurse, who will decide where the patients should go for further treatment.	
	• how to distribute equipment and supplies?	☐	☐	The materials management staff has an emergency supply distribution list to refer to during a disaster.	
	• who will notify the authorities of the disaster?	☐	☐	The chief security officer is responsible for reporting any disasters to state and local authorities as required by law.	
	• who will handle media attention?	☐	☐	The public relations staff is responsible for fielding all media inquiries and questions.	
	• how to handle a utility failure during an emergency?	☐	☐	The hospital has an agreement with a contractor to supply a water tanker, if needed; radios are available in the event of a telephone system failure.	

The JCAHO Mock Survey Made Simple, 1999 Edition

Checklist 23: The Seven Environment of Care Plans

Standard	Assessment Point	Yes	No	Example of Compliance	Notes
cont'd	• if you can provide chemical radioactive decontamination and isolation, if needed?	☐	☐	There is a decontamination shower and attached isolation room in the emergency department and outpatient area.	
Life Safety Management Plan					
EC.1.7 EC.2.6	Do you have a life safety management plan that describes • how the organization will meet the 1997 *Life Safety Code®*?	☐	☐	Your facility should meet all life safety requirements, such as having fire doors on each unit, no holes in your fire walls, and a sufficient number of emergency exits.	
	• when you will inspect, test, and perform preventative maintenance on the hospital's - fire alarms and detection systems? - circuits? - automatic fire extinguishing systems? - smoke control devices?	☐☐☐☐	☐☐☐☐	The hospital follows a fire safety inspection, testing, and preventative maintenance calendar.	
	• how to manage all life and fire safety problems?	☐	☐	During routine safety inspections, fire safety problems are identified and reported to the safety committee for investigation and resolution.	
	• how to ensure that all bed clothing, linens, blinds, draperies, curtains, trash cans, and furniture are fire safe?	☐	☐	The safety committee has developed criteria staff can use to gauge whether new items meet life safety standards.	

The JCAHO Mock Survey Made Simple, 1999 Edition

Checklist 23: The Seven Environment of Care Plans

Standard	Assessment Point	Yes	No	Example of Compliance	Notes
cont'd	• whether you maintain structural drawings of your buildings?	☐	☐	Blueprints for all buildings should be readily available in the facilities management office.	
	• when and how to implement Interim Life Safety Measures during construction and/or renovation?	☐	☐	During periods of construction and renovation, the facilities manager, along with other appropriate persons, such as security and biomedical engineering, develops a plan which will ensure that there are sufficient exits from each area and adequate fire extinguishing equipment and exit signs.	
	• how to teach staff about life safety management?	☐	☐	All employees are taught life safety procedures, such as how to use the hospital's fire alarm system, handle an evacuation, or contain a fire.	
	• how you will monitor at least one performance standard in the area of life safety?	☐	☐	The hospital monitors and evaluates employees' response to fire drills and reports these results to the safety committee.	
Equipment Management Plan					
🏃 EC.1.8 EC.2.7	Do you have an equipment management plan which describes • how the hospital will determine which pieces of equipment are to be included in the equipment management plan?	☐	☐	The hospital has developed assessment criteria designed to evaluate which materials in the hospital should be included in the equipment management plan; this individual has used the criteria to determine that the hospital's ventilators and dialysis machines are high risk and should be included in the equipment management plan, while the hospital's bedside tables do not meet the criteria and should be excluded from the plan.	

The JCAHO Mock Survey Made Simple, 1999 Edition

Checklist 23: The Seven Environment of Care Plans

Standard	Assessment Point	Yes	No	Example of Compliance	Notes
cont'd	• which pieces of equipment meet this criteria? • your preventative maintenance schedule for all the equipment included in your plan?	☐ ☐	☐ ☐	The hospital has developed an annual preventative maintenance schedule; staff who perform preventative maintenance sign off on your schedule to indicate that their work has been completed.	
	• how you will handle equipment recalls and/or alerts?	☐	☐	The hospital has identified who is responsible for handling equipment recalls or alerts, what steps these individuals should take, and how they should document their actions.	
	• how you comply with the Safe Medical Device Act?	☐	☐	The hospital's risk manager and biomedical engineer review and evaluate all potential device failures and document their actions.	
	• how you will handle all equipment related problems?	☐	☐	The hospital's biomedical engineer reports all equipment operator errors to the safety committee.	
	• how to handle equipment emergencies?	☐	☐	The hospital keeps Ambu bags near all ventilators in case of a power or equipment failure; the biomedical engineering's emergency number is posted near all equipment and at the nurses' station so that staff can quickly get help when a critical piece of equipment fails.	
	• how to teach staff to use all equipment, as applicable to their jobs?	☐	☐	The hospital teaches staff how to correctly and safely use equipment relative to the employee's job and how to handle and report equipment failures.	

The JCAHO Mock Survey Made Simple, 1999 Edition

Checklist 23: The Seven Environment of Care Plans

Standard	Assessment Point	Yes	No	Example of Compliance	Notes
cont'd	• how to monitor at least one performance standard for equipment management?	☐	☐	User errors are tracked and trended by the type of equipment and unit/area and the results are reported to safety committee.	

Utility Management Plan

Standard	Assessment Point	Yes	No	Example of Compliance	Notes
EC.1.9 EC.2.8	Do you have a utility management plan that describes how you will • determine which utilities and utility components should be included in your management program? • manage all of your utility systems? • evaluate and maintain your equipment? • handle emergency system failures? • determine the layout of each utility and the location of its control panels? • handle any problems with a utility? • provide an emergency power source that can maintain all of the hospital's essential functions, if needed? • teach staff how to manage the hospital's utilities as applicable to their jobs? • monitor at least one performance standard for utility management?	☐ ☐ ☐ ☐ ☐ ☐ ☐ ☐ ☐ ☐	☐ ☐ ☐ ☐ ☐ ☐ ☐ ☐ ☐ ☐	The hospital teaches employees the emergency procedures for shutting off a utility and reporting a utility problem or failure. The hospital monitors and evaluates all utility failures and reports their results to the safety committee.	

Checklist 23: The Seven Environment of Care Plans

Standard	Assessment Point	Yes	No	Example of Compliance	Notes
All Plans					
🏃 EC.1.3– EC.1.9 EC.2.2– EC.2.8	Do you evaluate the quality and effectiveness of each of your seven environment of care (EC) plans or programs at least annually?	☐	☐	The safety committee has appointed several small sub-groups to annually review and evaluate each of the seven EC plans; these sub-groups present their findings to the safety committee for final review and approval.	
	Do you report to the hospital board of directors at least quarterly on the status of the seven EC plans?	☐	☐	The chairperson of the safety committee prepares a summary report of the safety committee's activities and presents it to the medical executive committee and the board of directors each quarter.	
	Do the performance standards monitored by each plan include at least one monitor related to on of the following areas: • employee knowledge and skill? • employee participation? • emergencies and/or incidents? • monitoring and inspection activities? • inspection, testing, and preventative maintenance on equipment?	☐☐☐☐☐	☐☐☐☐☐		

CEO's Responsibilities 24

It's clear from the JCAHO standards that compliance begins with leadership, specifically with the direction and structure set forth by the chief executive officer (CEO). While the ultimate responsibility for the hospital rests with the governing body, these individuals delegate most of the operational and organizational details to the CEO. By the CEO's deed and example, he or she can be instrumental in ensuring that the hospital operates successfully, which will then translates into a successful JCAHO survey.

Checklist 24: CEO's Responsibilities

Standard	Assessment Point	Yes	No	Example of Compliance	Notes
✈ RI.1 RI.4	Do you develop, support, and implement policies that promote high ethical standards in your patient care and business practices?	☐	☐	A working mechanism, such as an ethics committee or trained team, is used to resolve ethical dilemmas; a conflict of interest policy is implemented at all levels of leadership; a patient representative program advocates patients' rights; these policies have been organized into a code of ethical behavior.	
PE.1–PE.1.5 TX.1.2 LD.2– LD.2.2 PI.1.1	Do you ensure that all members of the health care team collaborate to meet patients' needs?	☐	☐	An organization-wide Plan of Care describes all of the services the hospital provides and how they are related; medical staff members participate in interdisciplinary performance improvement teams; all patient assessment information is integrated into an interdisciplinary plan of care.	
CC.1–CC.8	Do you ensure that all patients have equal access to care and that all discharges and transfers are appropriate?	☐	☐	A utilization management program ensures that patients are treated in appropriate care settings and receive safe, effective discharge plans; the hospital has a policy to address denial-of-care decisions by insurers; transfers adhere to federal regulations for access to care.	
✈ LD.1 LD.4	Do you require leaders and staff to base their planning and improvement efforts on measured and analyzed data, whether the information is derived from something as broad-based as a community assessment or as specific as turn-around times for lab services?	☐	☐	New service proposals must be supported by data and information.	

The JCAHO Mock Survey Made Simple, 1999 Edition

Checklist 24: CEO's Responsibilities

Standard	Assessment Point	Yes	No	Example of Compliance	Notes
🏃 LD.1.1	Have you developed mission, vision, and values statements for the hospital?	☐	☐	Executive staff reviews the hospital's mission, vision, and values statements annually and uses them as a reference point for updating the strategic plan, capital expenditure list, and the budget.	
	Have you created strategic, operating, and financial plans to help you achieve these goals?	☐	☐		
🏃 LD.1.2	Have you communicated the hospital's mission, vision, and values statements to employees, medical staff, and volunteers?	☐	☐	The hospital's mission, vision, and values are the subject of management meeting(s) and departmental meetings and are explained to all employees in your internal newspaper.	
LD.3.3	Have you established open and effective lines of communication between the hospital, its staff, and customers?	☐	☐	CEO holds periodic "Town Meetings" with all staff; managers liaison with other providers in the community to look for opportunities to improve their service to the community.	
🏃 LD.4.1	Do you understand the basic tenets of "generic continuous quality improvement" and the specifics of the hospital's performance improvement (PI) plan?	☐	☐	You insist on analysis of data before approval of any performance improvement plans and coach other leaders to apply PI principles in their daily work.	
	Do you apply these principles in daily work?	☐	☐		
🏃 LD.4.3.2 PI.5	Can you speak intelligently about significant PI in the organization over the last 18 months?	☐	☐	You understand at least five of the hospital's key improvement projects well enough to explain why they were selected, what you hoped to achieve, how the "fix" was implemented, what the post measurements showed, and what "tweaking" had to be done before the plan was fully implemented; you can relate the hospital's PI plan to the JCAHO standards and can give a little history of how the organization's approach to PI has evolved over the years.	

The JCAHO Mock Survey Made Simple, 1999 Edition

Checklist 24: CEO's Responsibilities

Standard	Assessment Point	Yes	No	Example of Compliance	Notes
🏃 LD.4.3 LD.4.3.1	Do you require all senior leaders to play an active role in PI and coach their department managers to do the same?	☐	☐	You require senior leaders to report on their participation in PI activities in quarterly progress reports; leaders' participation in PI activities is reviewed in their annual performance evaluations.	
EC.1	Do you promote and implement policies requiring your hospital to be safe, clean, accessible, and attractive, according to your mission and any applicable state or federal regulations?	☐	☐	Environment of care manuals address all of these issues; safety reports are submitted to the governing body; a tour of the facility demonstrates compliance.	
🏃 HR.1 PI.5	Have you supported clear competency standards for hiring and retaining hospital employees and medical staff members?	☐	☐	Job descriptions and policies exist to help the hospital ensure it hires qualified staff; staff competency is periodically reviewed.	
HR.3.1	Have you created staff training and educational opportunities for everyone in the hospital?	☐	☐	The annual budget has reasonable allowance for in-house training of staff and tuition reimbursement for continuing education.	
🏃 IM.1	Have you helped to develop the hospital's information management (IM) plan?	☐	☐	A steering committee, including the CEO or his/her delegates, develops an IM plan that is consistent with the hospital's scope, vision, and complexity of services; your capital expenditures plan provides the resources necessary to implement the IM plan.	
	Have you ensured that it is consistent with the hospital's strategic and capital expenditures plans?	☐	☐		
🏃 IM.2	Have you established clear expectations for the confidentiality and security of all data and medical records?	☐	☐	Human resources policies address the seriousness of breaches of confidentiality; IM procedure requires users to sign an acknowledgement of the policy.	

The JCAHO Mock Survey Made Simple, 1999 Edition

Checklist 24: CEO's Responsibilities

STANDARD	ASSESSMENT POINT	YES	NO	EXAMPLE OF COMPLIANCE	NOTES
✈ IM.7	Do you ensure that every patient who is examined and treated has a complete, accurate, and timely medical record?	☐	☐	Working with the medical staff, the CEO enforces policies requiring all records to be completed within 30 days of discharge.	
GO.1–GO.2.6	Do you provide the governing board with all of the information it needs to fulfill its duties?	☐	☐	The CEO provides the governing board with reports on hospital safety, staff competence, PI activities, compliance with applicable regulations, strategic plans, and the hospital's finances.	
MA.3 LD.4.4	Do you operate a fiscally responsible organization? Are you responsible and accountable for its efficiency and quality of services?	☐	☐	Managers are required to submit a monthly or quarterly budget compliance report along with goals and progress reports; sufficient resources are allocated for performance improvement activities.	
MA.4	Have you established clear processes for the utilization and conservation of human, operating, capital, and space resources?	☐	☐	A multidisciplinary committee reviews requests for new positions, service enhancements, and capital requests.	
✈ MS.1–MS.4	Do you offer the medical staff the guidance and resources it needs to develop and implement its bylaws and properly conduct its business?	☐	☐	A full-time medical staff coordinator is provided for in the budget; the CEO attends the medical executive committee meetings and reports on information pertinent to the medical staff; the CEO meets weekly with the president of the medical staff to discuss all issues of joint concern.	

Department Managers' Responsibilities 25

With the introduction of the JCAHO's integrated standards, life became more complex for department managers. Originally, they were responsible for complying with only one chapter in the *Comprehensive Accreditation Manual for Hospitals (CAMH)*, but when the JCAHO reshuffled all of the standards in the *CAMH*, these managers' responsibilities changed. Now they were required to wade through all of the standards and determine which ones pertained to their areas, and which didn't.

Since this overhaul of the *CAMH*, the JCAHO's basic requirements haven't changed very much. You can expect JCAHO surveyors to want to see that your department managers foster an atmosphere of collaboration, communication, and continuous performance improvement in their respective areas. The following checklist presents the key requirements pertaining to medical and administrative department managers and should be used to test their knowledge of these issues.

Checklist 25: Department Managers' Responsibilities

Standard	Assessment Point	Yes	No	Example of Compliance	Notes
❖ RI.1	Do you know how to resolve patient care ethical dilemmas in your department?	☐	☐	The hospital has an ethics team which has been trained to evaluate and resolve ethical questions; these individuals are available for consultation 365 days per year.	
❖ RI.1.2 RI.1.3 RI.2	Are you familiar with the hospital's policies on • organ donation? • withholding or withdrawing treatment? • participating in research or investigational studies? • care at the end of life? • securing religious or spiritual counseling? • handling a patient's refusal of treatment?	☐☐☐ ☐☐☐	☐☐☐ ☐☐☐	All of these policies are documented in the organization's administrative manual, which is distributed to every department.	
RI.1.2.1	Do you know how to obtain informed consent?	☐	☐	There is an informed consent manual which explains the informed consent process; the hospital's informed consent policy requires staff to explain to the patient the proposed treatment, its alternatives, any major risks, the name of the person who will perform the procedure, and the patient's right to refuse treatment, particularly in regard to the use of research protocols.	
RI.1.4	Do you understand how to inform patients of their rights?	☐	☐	Patient's rights are printed in the patient handbook and distributed to all patients; summaries of all patient's rights are posted in patient waiting rooms.	

Checklist 25: Department Managers' Responsibilities

Standard	Assessment Point	Yes	No	Example of Compliance	Notes
🏃 RI.1.3.4	Do you know how to handle a patient or family member's complaint?	☐	☐	The hospital has patient representatives who advocate for patients when they have problems; these patient representatives ensure that each problem is investigated, resolved, and recorded; managers must address complaints in their departments; serious incidents are reported according to state and federal requirements.	
🏃 RI.4	Have you explained the hospital's code of ethics to staff?	☐	☐	The hospital's code of ethics is included in the administrative manual. It states that the organization's goals are to deliver excellent patient care and operate ethically and with integrity.	
PF.4–PF.4.2	Do you encourage staff to develop interdisciplinary patient education programs and materials?	☐	☐	All educational programs and materials are developed under the direction of an interdisciplinary work group.	
PF.4–PF.4.2	As you develop your budget, do you allot resources to support patient and family education?	☐	☐	The department budgets expenses for developing new patient and family educational materials each year.	
CC.4	Do you encourage staff to work with other disciplines as they transition patients from one setting to the next?	☐	☐	All staff have attended an educational program that encourages them to view the hospital's services from the patient's viewpoint and stresses the importance of working together to eliminate barriers to seamless service.	

The JCAHO Mock Survey Made Simple, 1999 Edition

Checklist 25: Department Managers' Responsibilities

Standard	Assessment Point	Yes	No	Example of Compliance	Notes
✪ CC.6	Have you established mechanisms that will help ease patients and their families through your organization?	☐	☐	All patients scheduled for elective orthopedic surgery are required to have a home assessment prior to admission, which allows rehab services to plan to use adaptive techniques or to refer the patient to post-hospital services, such as home care.	
CC.6	As you develop new services, do you consider how they will fit into the hospital's continuum of care?	☐	☐	A new freestanding cancer center was designed to handle all of the cancer patient's primary needs at one site and includes laboratory, radiology, pharmacy, radiation therapy, and oncology services.	
✪ PI.1	Can you describe the basics of your hospital's performance improvement (PI) plan, such as • what is measured in your area?	☐	☐	Each department measures high volume, high risk, problem prone processes and outcomes, as well as customer satisfaction.	
	• how data is assessed?	☐	☐	Assessment tools such as run charts, control charts, histograms, and Pareto charts are used to assess data.	
	• how issues are selected for improvement?	☐	☐	When an assessment of a process indicates that its performance is not acceptable, a recommendation for improvement is made to the PI committee; the committee may also recommend improvements based on its review of submitted data; the committee has developed prioritization criteria.	

The JCAHO Mock Survey Made Simple, 1999 Edition

Checklist 25: Department Managers' Responsibilities

Standard	Assessment Point	Yes	No	Example of Compliance	Notes
cont'd	• what model is used for improvement?	☐	☐	The hospital uses a modified version of the 10 step model to guide all of its PI activities.	
	• how PI activities are communicated?	☐	☐	PI success stories are reported in the organization's internal newspaper; the status of all PI efforts are summarized and reported to the PI oversight committee, senior executives, and the board of trustees.	
	• who is responsible for overseeing improvements?	☐	☐	Leadership is responsible for assessing and improving services; staff are responsible for developing improvement suggestions and bringing them to their manager's attention; the ultimate responsibility for PI rests with the governing body.	
PI.3 PI.4	Do you incorporate the principles of PI into your department's daily work?	☐	☐	Results of monitoring activities are posted in the manager's office and shared with staff at monthly staff meetings; managers ask the staff to assess the quality of their department's processes and determine if they can be improved.	
PI.3.1	Do you discuss PI at staff meetings or have some other mechanism for collecting staff views about PI?	☐	☐	Meeting minutes outline staff suggestions for PI opportunities.	
PI.5	Do you evaluate the success of your contributions to the hospital's PI program?	☐	☐	During annual departmental evaluations, managers review their personal contributions to the hospital's PI program and ask staff how they think their department can be improved in the coming year.	

Checklist 25: Department Managers' Responsibilities

Standard	Assessment Point	Yes	No	Example of Compliance	Notes
LD.1 LD.1.1	Does your department's PI plan support the hospital-wide mission and vision?	☐	☐	Key goals in your department's PI plan were developed in direct response to the hospital's mission and vision, and further the goals of the hospital-wide PI plan.	
🏃 LD.1.3.3	Do you assess the needs of your department's internal and external customers?	☐	☐	The laboratory manager uses focus groups to assess the changing needs of the hospital's ambulatory units; the utilization management department surveyed managed care companies for common data needs to ensure they were collecting the right data efficiently.	
🏃 LD.2.2	Do you coordinate and integrate your department's services with those in other departments?	☐	☐	Each department manager routinely consults with other stakeholders, such as other managers, medical staff members, and community agencies, and counsels staff to do the same; there are no barriers to cooperation between departments.	
LD.2.3	Is your area of responsibility organized and staffed appropriately?	☐	☐	Schedules and staffing records, policies and procedures all reflect adequate staffing in the organization.	
🏃 EC.2 EC.2.1	Have you trained staff on safety issues such as • fire safety? • life safety? • infection control? • the handling of hazardous materials, hazardous waste, and equipment and utility failures? • disaster preparedness? • evacuation procedures?	☐☐☐☐ ☐☐	☐☐☐☐ ☐☐	Managers discuss the hospital's procedures for each of these issues with staff; staff are oriented to these safety issues at the time of hire and in annual refresher sessions.	

The JCAHO Mock Survey Made Simple, 1999 Edition

Checklist 25: Department Managers' Responsibilities

Standard	Assessment Point	Yes	No	Example of Compliance	Notes
EC.3 EC.3.2	Have you reduced safety risks to your staff?	☐	☐	Documentation indicates that department managers purchased new hazardous waste bags after they discovered that the previous bags were too flimsy.	
EC.3.1	Do you know how to file an occurrence report?	☐	☐	Hospital records indicate that managers have filed occurrence reports in the past.	
EC.3.1	Have you taught staff how to file occurrence reports?	☐	☐	Staff are taught how to file occurrence reports in new employee orientations and in annual refresher seminars.	
EC.3.3	Do you budget for departmental safety improvements?	☐	☐	Each department's budget for the upcoming year reflects the increased costs of safer and more durable biohazard bags.	
HR.1	Have you developed job descriptions for each staff member?	☐	☐	Departmental files contain job descriptions for each position; staff are familiar with their job descriptions and each has his or her own copy.	
HR.2	Do you consider potential changes in staffing needs when developing your department's budget?	☐	☐	Department managers consider the potential costs of increased patient volumes, service improvements, and compliance with regulatory requirements as they develop their budgets.	
✵	Do you ensure that each employee receives an initial and annual evaluation of his or her competency based on his or her job description?	☐	☐	Departmental files indicate that the staff's performance is evaluated each year; competency checklists are used to assess staff competency.	
HR.3	Do these annual evaluations address age-specific competencies?	☐	☐		

The JCAHO Mock Survey Made Simple, 1999 Edition

Checklist 25: Department Managers' Responsibilities

Standard	Assessment Point	Yes	No	Example of Compliance	Notes
HR.3.1	Do you encourage staff to participate in self-development activities?	☐	☐	Each department's budget reflects staff training expenses; performance evaluations include comments on each staff member's potential for advancement.	
	Do you promote career advancement for staff?	☐	☐		
HR.4	Do you orient and train your staff?	☐	☐	Departmental budgets indicate that money has been allotted for orientation and training in departmental procedures.	
IM.1.1.2	Did you help to develop the organization's information management (IM) plan?	☐	☐	Each department manager helped generate the framework for the hospital's IM plan by completing an information needs survey and participating in a priority setting session.	
✈ IM.1.1	Are you familiar with the hospital's IM plan?	☐	☐	Each department manager understands the hospital's current IM capabilities and how they will be improved over the next two years.	
IM.4	Do you know the difference between data and information?	☐	☐	Each department manager can give examples of the performance data collected in his or her area, such as waiting times or delays in first doses of antibiotics, and how that data is converted into meaningful information by using analysis tools.	

Checklist 25: Department Managers' Responsibilities

Standard	Assessment Point	Yes	No	Example of Compliance	Notes
IM.7.2 IM.8 IM.9–IM.9.2	Can you demonstrate how your department uses and obtains • patient-specific data? • patient-specific information? • aggregated data? • aggregated information? • current literature?	☐☐☐☐☐	☐☐☐☐☐	Managers use this data or information as applicable to their areas of expertise; patient-specific information needed for diagnosis and treatment is gathered promptly; aggregated data and its resulting information is used to develop budgets; information in journals and other literature is used to plan a new service.	
✈ IM.10	Do you know which external, interactive, and comparative databases are used by the hospital?	☐	☐	The hospital participates in the Maryland Hospital Association Program as well as the JCAHO's IMS program.	
IM.2	Have your staff been taught how to use the hospital's information systems?	☐	☐	All new staff are taught how to use the hospital's information systems before they begin their duties; experienced staff are taught how to use new applications; the hospital assesses staff's understanding of its information systems and determines who needs to be retrained.	
IM.2.1	If your department uses passwords, are they confidential and changed periodically?	☐	☐	Each employee is assigned a password at training and is asked to sign a statement agreeing to keep that password confidential; each password is changed every six months.	
IM.7 IM.7.1.1 IM.7.1.3.1	If your department handles medical records, do your staff understand • who is authorized to make entries? • how to make entries in the record? • if any electronic signatures can be accepted? • how to use your approved abbreviation list?	☐☐☐☐	☐☐☐☐	New employees are taught how to maintain the medical record; medical record policies are reviewed periodically during staff meetings.	

Checklist 25: Department Managers' Responsibilities

Standard	Assessment Point	Yes	No	Example of Compliance	Notes
IM.1.1.2	Do you consider your department's information needs as you develop your budget and capital requests?	☐	☐	Your department budgets for any information costs not included in the hospital-wide information management budget, such as the need for minor and capital equipment like replacement hardware or new software upgrades.	
IC.1 IC.1.1	Do you work with the infection control (IC) department to develop departmental IC policies and procedures?	☐	☐	Departmental IC policies are reviewed annually with the IC department and are submitted to the IC committee for approval.	
IC.4	Have your staff been oriented to and trained on the hospital's IC policies and procedures?	☐	☐	All new employees are oriented to basic universal precautions and hand washing procedures and are trained on their department's specific infection control policies during the first two weeks of employment.	
Managers responsible for patient care areas:					
PE.1 PE.2	Do you understand the hospital's patient assessment policies and procedures?	☐	☐	Patients are assessed within eight hours of admission or at the time of each ambulatory visit; MDs, RNs, NPs, CRNAs, dietitians, physical therapists, occupational therapists, speech therapists, respiratory therapists, and child life specialists participate in each assessment, as needed; reassessment is required if the patient experiences significant changes; acute patients must be reassessed at a minimum of every three days.	

The JCAHO Mock Survey Made Simple, 1999 Edition

Checklist 25: Department Managers' Responsibilities

Standard	Assessment Point	Yes	No	Example of Compliance	Notes
TX.1	Do you know how to develop an interdisciplinary care plan?	☐	☐	Each care plan is developed according to a patient's interdisciplinary assessment; the attending physician and primary nurse develop the care plan; information system tools and multidisciplinary rounds support this process.	
✣ TX.7.1.1	Do you support appropriate use of restraint and/or seclusion by • reviewing and revising, if needed, your department's restraint and seclusion policies and procedures? • evaluating alternatives to restraint or seclusion? • maintaining appropriate staffing levels to minimize the need for restraint and/or to ensure that staff are available to perform checks when restraint is used? • orienting and training staff on restraint and seclusion policies and procedures? • educating patients and their families about restraint and/or seclusion when it is needed?	☐ ☐ ☐☐ ☐ ☐	☐ ☐ ☐☐ ☐ ☐	Restraint use in non-psychiatric areas is intensively monitored; restraint use has been reduced by relocating patients needing special attention closer to the nurse's station, by using family sitters, and by gauging whether medications contribute to behavioral problems.	
✣ HR.6	Are you familiar with the hospital's policy on handling employees' requests to not participate in patient care because of their cultural values or religious beliefs?	☐	☐	This policy is in your administrative manual; you document all such requests and their outcomes in the employee's folder.	

Medical Staff Leaders' Responsibilities 26

The JCAHO requires medical staff members to familiarize themselves with a number of its key requirements, such as those for performance improvement, patient assessment, infection control, care of the patient, and information management standards. And it's up to medical staff leaders to ensure that their staff is compliant. By using this checklist, these leaders can identify the JCAHO's key medical staff requirements and pinpoint which areas are strengths for their organization, and which are weaknesses.

Checklist 28. Medical Staff Leaders' Responsibilities

Standard	Assessment Point	Yes	No	Example of Compliance	Notes
⚹ PE.1.6.1 PE.1.6.1.1	Do medical staff members complete legible histories and physicals (H&Ps) for each patient within 24 hours of admission or within 30 days prior to admission? *Note: Medicare requires an update to any H&P older than 7 days.*	☐	☐	A policy states that patients who had H&Ps completed by their primary care physicians within 30 days prior to surgery should have their H&Ps sent to the hospital before surgery and included in their medical record.	
⚹ TX.3.1 TX.4.1 TX.5 TX.7 TX.7.1.3.11 RI.2	Are you involved in developing • the hospital's medications list? • nutritional therapy plans for nutritionally high risk patients? • pre-operative assessment guidelines? • restraint and seclusion policies and procedures? • organ donation policies and procedures?	☐☐ ☐☐ ☐	☐☐ ☐☐ ☐	Medical staff leaders participate on the pharmacy and therapeutics committee to develop the hospital formulary; the anesthesia department develops anesthesia guidelines and obtains the medical executive committee's (MEC) approval.	
PI.1	Do all medical staff members understand the hospital's approach to performance improvement (PI)?	☐	☐	As part of each clinical department's monthly or quarterly meeting, the chief provides some basic information on the hospital's approach to PI; physicians who join quality improvement teams are educated on the hospital's chosen PI model.	
EC.1.3– EC.1.9	Do all medical staff members understand the hospital's fire, internal and external disaster, and hazardous materials management plans?	☐	☐	All medical staff members know the hospital's emergency codes, the locations of all exits, and all emergency numbers; all medical staff members know how and where to respond to each emergency code.	
IM.1.1.2	Do you help assess the hospital's information needs and select appropriate information technologies to meet those needs?	☐	☐	Representatives from the medical staff participated in the hospital task force to evaluate the hospital's information management needs.	

The JCAHO Mock Survey Made Simple, 1999 Edition

227

Checklist 26: Medical Staff Leaders' Responsibilities

Standard	Assessment Point	Yes	No	Example of Compliance	Notes
IM.3.2.1.1	Do medical staff members participate in medical record reviews?	☐	☐	Physicians participate in the hospital's medical records quality committee and help review the results of medical records, perform individual case review when needed, and follow up with attending physicians with delinquent medical records.	
🏃 IM.7.3.2.1	Do all medical staff members dictate operative notes the day a procedure is performed?	☐	☐	The medical staff has a policy that requires an operative note to be either written or dictated immediately following surgery. If not transcribed immediately, there must be a written note.	
🏃 IM.7.7	Has the medical staff approved policies and procedures regarding the signing of verbal orders?	☐	☐	The medical staff has a policy that requires all verbal orders to be signed within 24 hours.	
IC.6.1.1	Have you developed reporting lines between the infection control program and the medical staff?	☐	☐	The infection control committee sends written reports on infection rates to the medical staff quality committee.	
🏃 MS.1– MS.3.1.6	Does the medical staff report to the board of directors?	☐	☐	Recommendations from the MEC go to the board of directors for approval; various medical staff activities are reported to the board through a quality improvement committee.	
MS.4.2.1.1 MS.4.2.1.2	Do you oversee and manage all clinical and administrative activities in your department?	☐	☐	The department chief reviews the results of peer reviews to evaluate the quality of care the department provides; the chief supports the department administratively by monitoring its budget and requesting new equipment and services.	

228

The JCAHO Mock Survey Made Simple, 1999 Edition

Checklist 26: Medical Staff Leaders' Responsibilities

Standard	Assessment Point	Yes	No	Example of Compliance	Notes
🏃 MS.4.2.1.3	Do you evaluate the performance of individual practitioners within your department?	☐	☐	Before making a recommendation to appoint or reappoint a physician to the department, you review the results of departmental monitoring and evaluations of the practitioner.	
🏃 MS.4.2.1.4 MS.4.2.1.5 MS.5.13	Do you recommend which members of your department should be reappointed or reprivileged?	☐	☐	Before making a privileging recommendation to the MEC, you review and evaluate the results of all departmental peer reviews, any lodged complaints and problems, and each individual's compliance with medical staff bylaws.	
MS.4.2.1.6	Do you recommend how the hospital can best access services that patients need but the hospital does not provide?	☐	☐	If your hospital doesn't offer radiation oncology, the medical staff chief may recommend that the hospital should contract for those services with a nearby radiation oncology facility.	
MS.4.2.1.7 MS.4.2.1.8 LD.2.1 LD.2.3	Do you ensure that your department integrates its services with the rest of the hospital?	☐	☐	The surgical chief works with the anesthesia and nursing departments to ensure that patients receive excellent post-procedure care.	
MS.4.2.1.10 MS.4.2.1.11 LD.2.4 LD.2.5	Do you determine how many support staff your department needs and what the qualifications are for these positions?	☐	☐	The medical director of the cath lab, with the department manager, determines how many support staff members the department needs based upon the volume of performed procedures.	
MS.4.2.1.12 LD.2.6	Do you ensure that the quality of your department's services continually improves?	☐	☐	As a result of a study on post-surgical infection rates in your department, the use of a new skin prep is recommended.	

The JCAHO Mock Survey Made Simple, 1999 Edition

Checklist 26: Medical Staff Leaders' Responsibilities

Standard	Assessment Point	Yes	No	Example of Compliance	Notes
MS.4.2.1.13 LD.2.7	Do you maintain quality controls where applicable, such as in the operating suite or the laboratory?	☐	☐	The chief of pathology ensures that all equipment and machinery is inspected and tested regularly.	
MS.4.2.1.14 LD.2.8	Do you ensure that all department support staff receive appropriate orientation and training?	☐	☐	The chief of radiology sends all of his support staff to the hospital's annual educational and training programs on fire safety and infection control.	
MS.4.2.1.15 LD.2.9	Do you make recommendations for space planning when appropriate?	☐	☐	If the radiology department plans to bring in a new MRI, the chief of radiology should assess the department's available space, determine how this new piece of equipment can be accommodated, and make his or her recommendations to the administration and/or board of directors.	
MS.5.1.1 MS.5.16	Does the entire medical staff comply with all medical staff and governing board bylaws, rules, regulations, and policies?	☐	☐	A review of patient charts proves that the medical staff documents patients' H&Ps within 24 hours, as required by the medical staff bylaws.	
MS.6.2	Do all inpatients receive their H&Ps from a member of the medical staff or a privileged licensed independent practitioner (LIP)?	☐	☐	The H&P of a patient recently seen by his or her primary care physician is added to the hospital's chart when the patient is admitted for same-day surgery.	
MS.5.10 MS.5.10.1	Does the hospital have each member of the medical staff's written consent to obtain and review documents and records pertinent to the appointment and privileging process?	☐	☐	The hospital obtained a signed statement from the medical staff applicant at the time of his or her appointment or reappointment.	

The JCAHO Mock Survey Made Simple, 1999 Edition

Checklist 26: Medical Staff Leaders' Responsibilities

Standard	Assessment Point	Yes	No	Example of Compliance	Notes
MS.5.10.2	Do all medical staff members provide their patients with ongoing care?	☐	☐	When appointed to the medical staff, each physician signs a written statement acknowledging that he or she is responsible for the continuous care of all patients admitted to his or her service.	
🏃 MS.6.3	Do medical staff members define which ambulatory and outpatient areas require an H&P?	☐	☐	The medical staff has defined that H&Ps are required in the ambulatory surgery unit, but not in outpatient treatment areas.	
🏃 MS.6.8	Do all patients receive consistently high quality care throughout the hospital?	☐	☐	Orthopedic surgeons and podiatrists must meet the same privileging criteria to operate on a patient's foot.	
MS.7 MS.7.1	Does the hospital sponsor continuing medical education for all physicians and LIPs with delineated clinical privileges?	☐	☐	The hospital offers continuing medical education credit for attendance at an educational program focused on the treatment and management of patients with tuberculosis.	
🏃 MS.8 MS.8.1 MS.8.2	Is the medical staff involved in performance improvement activities affecting areas such as • patient assessment and treatment? • medication use and blood use? • operative procedures? • clinical outcomes? • patient and family education? • care coordination? • medical records completion?	☐☐☐☐☐☐☐	☐☐☐☐☐☐☐	The clinical chief reviews aggregate data on the results of drug and blood use and looks for patterns, trends, and PI opportunities; physicians help develop clinical pathways.	

The JCAHO Mock Survey Made Simple, 1999 Edition

Checklist 26: Medical Staff Leaders' Responsibilities

Standard	Assessment Point	Yes	No	Example of Compliance	Notes
MS.8.3 MS.8.4	Do medical staff members use the results of PI activities to improve the care the hospital offers?	☐	☐	The medical staff chief reviews all readmissions quarterly and uses this information to make re-appointment decisions.	
	Do you use the results of PI activities to make re-appointment decisions?	☐	☐		
🏃 MS.8.5.1–MS.8.5.3	Have you established criteria to determine when an autopsy is needed and how to notify the patient's attending physician?	☐	☐	The MEC has approved autopsy request criteria that meet both legal and clinical autopsy requirements.	

Line Staff's Responsibilities 27

Your line staff should be able to demonstrate that they understand a number of basic JCAHO requirements in areas such as patient rights and organization ethics, performance improvement, leadership, environment of care, human resources, information management, patient assessment, infection control, care of the patient, patient and family education, and continuum of care.

Give the following checklist to your line staff to familiarize them with pertinent JCAHO requirements, or use it to stimulate discussion in staff meetings. While we have supplied examples of compliance for each question, many of these questions will require hospital-specific answers. Managers should review these issues, such as the hospital's mission, with their staff.

Consider holding contests to encourage staff to study these requirements, and offer prizes to everyone who knows the right answers. This creative approach to survey preparation makes the task of teaching JCAHO requirements to hundreds of staff a little less onerous for the survey coordinator.

Checklist 27. EMS Staff's Responsibilities

STANDARD	ASSESSMENT POINT	YES	NO	EXAMPLE OF COMPLIANCE	NOTES
For all staff:					
RI.1	Do you know what to do if you have an ethical question regarding the care of a patient?	☐	☐	Speak to your manager and ask his or her advice on how to address the issue.	
🏃 RI.1.1	Do you know, or know where to find, a list of patient's rights and responsibilities?	☐	☐	A list of patient's rights and responsibilities is usually located in the patient handbook or posted in admitting registration areas or on placards in patient rooms.	
🏃 RI.1.3	Do you understand how to • maintain patient confidentiality? • respect patients' privacy? • protect patients' security? • handle patients' complaints or requests for pastoral/spiritual counseling? • help patients who need communication assistance?	☐☐☐☐ ☐	☐☐☐☐ ☐	This information is typically covered in new employee orientations and updated annually during competency evaluations; there is usually an employee handbook or personnel policy manual to which you can refer for specific information on your institution.	
🏃 PI.3.2.6	Do you know where you should bring a suggestion for improvement?	☐	☐	Put your suggestion in the hospital's suggestion box; take it to your manager; submit it to the quality resources department.	
🏃 PI.5	Can you think of one or two improvements made during the last year in your area?	☐	☐	Your manager has discussed process improvements in your area during staff meetings; hospital-wide improvements have been reported in the hospital newsletter and during "Quality Week."	

The JCAHO Mock Survey Made Simple, 1999 Edition

235

Checklist 27: Line Staff's Responsibilities

Standard	Assessment Point	Yes	No	Example of Compliance	Notes
PI.5	Do you know what measures are collected and assessed in your area?	☐	☐	Your department collects measures on patient satisfaction, use of restraint, medication errors, patient falls, or other high volume, high risk, problem prone areas; your manager reports the results of these measures at staff meetings.	
✸ LD.1.2	Do you know your hospital's mission, vision, and values?	☐	☐	Staff know the hospital's mission, vision, and values or know where to find written copies of them; some hospitals print their mission, vision, and values on the back of all ID badges or in the hospital newspaper.	
✸ EC.2.1	Can you describe • any safety risks in your workplace and what steps you've taken to reduce or eliminate them? • how you would file an incident or occurrence report? • what your responsibilities are if there is a fire in the hospital or in your area? • the location of fire alarms? • your role in the hospital's evacuation procedure? • how to minimize security risks? • how to report security incidents? • how to safely handle, store, and dispose of hazardous wastes or materials? • how to report and manage hazardous spills or exposures? • the location of MSDSs?	☐ ☐ ☐ ☐ ☐☐ ☐☐☐ ☐ ☐	☐ ☐ ☐ ☐ ☐☐ ☐☐☐ ☐ ☐	All of this information should be located in your department's environment of care manual; your manager should be able to provide you with this safety information.	

Checklist 27: Line Staff's Responsibilities

Standard	Assessment Point	Yes	No	Example of Compliance	Notes
cont'd	• your role and responsibility during a disaster drill or true emergency? • the proper procedure for operating equipment in your area and reporting malfunctioning equipment? • what to do in case of equipment failure? • what to do in and how to report a power outage or other utility failure? • the location and use of emergency shut-offs, such as oxygen? • who to contact in case of an emergency?	☐ ☐ ☐☐ ☐ ☐	☐ ☐ ☐☐ ☐ ☐		
HR.4 HR.4.2	Have you been taught how to use the hospital's information systems, as pertinent to your job?	☐	☐	Unit secretaries are taught how to enter orders and results into the hospital's information system during their orientation.	
✶	Have you been oriented to your duties?	☐	☐	Staff are typically oriented to hospital-wide and department-specific issues during the first two to four weeks of employment.	
HR.4.2	Have you received job-specific training, if necessary?	☐	☐		
✶ HR.5	Is your competency evaluated periodically and based on your job description?	☐	☐	Annual performance evaluations based on your job description are held around your date of hire anniversary.	
✶ HR.6	Do you know what to do if you feel that you cannot participate in the care and treatment of a patient due to your religious belief or cultural values?	☐	☐	Policies and procedures on this topic are discussed during orientation; managers are available to discuss this issue with staff members.	

Checklist 27: Line Staff's Responsibilities

STANDARD	ASSESSMENT POINT	YES	NO	EXAMPLE OF COMPLIANCE	NOTES
✵ IM.2.3	If you use passwords, have you been instructed never to share the password with others?	☐	☐	Passwords are never shared and they are changed quarterly as an additional safeguard.	
✵ IM.2.3	If you work with patients' medical records, do you understand that all patient information must be confidential?	☐	☐	This policy is discussed at all employee orientations.	
IM.3 IM.3.1	Do you understand the need to adhere to data definitions and approved abbreviations in the medical record and other databases?	☐	☐	To enhance communication and safeguard the integrity of information, all staff are taught how to properly use and enter data according to the hospital's data definitions and abbreviations.	
✵ IC.4	Can you demonstrate knowledge of • universal precautions? • good hand washing technique? • all infection control policies relative to your work area?	☐☐☐	☐☐☐	Infection control basics are discussed during employees' hospital-wide orientation; infection control policies and procedures are located in each department.	
For patient caregivers only:					
✵ PE.1 TX.1–TX.1.3	Do you assess patients' care needs and develop corresponding care plans?	☐	☐	The hospital has an interdisciplinary process designed to synthesize all patient assessment information into patient care plans.	
✵ PE.1 TX.1–TX.1.3	Do you understand your role in implementing the plan of care and what policies and procedures you must follow?	☐	☐	The patient care assistant carries out vital patient care duties, as delegated by the RN, that do not require a licensed professional; licensed professionals assess, develop care plans for, treat, and educate patients.	

The JCAHO Mock Survey Made Simple, 1999 Edition

Checklist 27: Line Staff's Responsibilities

Standard	Assessment Point	Yes	No	Example of Compliance	Notes
TX.3.3 TX.4.7 TX.7 TX.7.4 PE.1.13 PE.2 PE.4	Do you know where procedure manuals are located, and whom you should consult if you cannot find an answer in the manual?	☐	☐	All manuals are located at the nurses' station; procedural questions not addressed in the procedure manual are directed to managers or supervisors.	
🏃 TX.7.1– TX.7.1.3.3	Have you been oriented and trained on the appropriate use of restraint?	☐	☐	All caregivers are oriented to the proper and limited use of restraint; all caregivers review restraint cases to determine if there are alternatives to restraint.	
🏃 PF.4 PF.4.1	Do you understand your role in patient and family education?	☐	☐	All RNs are expected to teach the patient and his or her family the skills/information needed to maintain and improve the patient's health.	
CC.5	Do you understand how your role fits within the continuum of care?	☐	☐	A discharge planner's role is to help caregivers develop a safe, effective discharge plan that will allow the patient to proceed to the next level of care as efficiently as possible; discharge is addressed from day one through the assessment so that the patient and family members always think about the post-hospital phase of care and aren't faced with any surprises or emergencies at the end of treatment.	

The JCAHO Mock Survey Made Simple, 1999 Edition

Related Products from Opus Communications, The Greeley Education Company, and The Greeley Company

NEWSLETTERS

Briefings on JCAHO

At over 3,700 hospitals nationwide, *Briefings on JCAHO* is the respected voice of authority for practical, independent guidance on succeeding in the accreditation process. Whether you're new to the survey game or are a seasoned professional, each issue offers quick reading and "how-to" advice on meeting JCAHO standards and tips and information that would otherwise cost dearly in consulting fees and research.

Some free subscriber benefits include the following:

- "BOJ Talk"—our Internet discussion group where readers can network with their peers; and
- Fax Express—whatever news happens that just can't wait, subscribers receive the pertinent information by fax so they'll always be the first to know.

Briefings on JCAHO: On-line

This restricted-access "Extranet site" allows an unlimited number of people at your facility to view and use BOJ at the same time. *Briefings on JCAHO* is the respected voice of authority for practical, independent guidance on succeeding in the accreditation process at over 3,700 hospitals nationwide. Each newsletter offers quick reading and "how-to" advice on meeting JCAHO standards. *Briefings on JCAHO: On-line* includes the text of articles, but no graphs or special reports. Subscribers to this on-line version will still receive a copy of the printed version of the monthly newsletter, as well as one printed copy of our special reports.

Briefings on JCAHO/AAAHC: Ambulatory Care

This monthly publication reports the activities of the ambulatory care accreditors: the Joint Commission on Accreditation of Healthcare Organizations (JCAHO) and the Accreditation Association for Ambulatory Health Care (AAAHC). It illustrates exactly what to do to pass a survey and gain accreditation so that organizations are known for quality and can affiliate with other delivery systems. With *Briefings on JCAHO/AAAHC: Ambulatory Care*, you'll learn how to prevent and correct problems and avoid JCAHO Type I recommendations. You'll also learn how to effectively balance an ever-increasing workload with compliance efforts.

Some free subscriber benefits include the following:

- "BOJ Talk"—our Internet discussion group where readers can network with their peers; and
- Fax Express—whatever news happens that just can't wait, subscribers receive the pertinent information by fax so they'll always be the first to know.

Briefings on Hospital Safety

Briefings on Hospital Safety advises hospital safety committees on how to meet the challenges of effective safety management. It provides safety committees with crucial information and offers guidance on how to improve safety in a hospital by preventing costly problems before they happen. All of the regulators are covered: JCAHO, OSHA, EPA, NFPA, FDA, and NRC.

Some free subscriber benefits include the following:

- "BHS Talk"—our Internet discussion group where readers can network with their peers; and
- Fax Express—whatever news happens that just can't wait, subscribers receive the pertinent information by fax so they'll always be the first to know.

Health Care Human Resources Alert

This monthly newsletter has everything readers need to make their job more manageable and time-efficient. From "how-to" articles to breaking news, *Health Care Human Resources Alert* keeps subscribers current on the latest rules and regulations and helps tailor their compliance program to meet tough government standards. It also enables readers to meet JCAHO standards and the challenges of privileging and credentialing allied health professionals.

Some free subscriber benefits include the following:

- "HR Talk"—our Internet discussion group where readers can network with their peers; and
- Fax Express—whatever news happens that just can't wait, subscribers receive the pertinent information by fax so they'll always be the first to know.

Long-Term Care Survey Monitor

Published monthly, *Long-Term Care Survey Monitor* helps you wade through the confusion and prepares them to meet the challenges of long-term and subacute care accreditation. You'll discover the latest industry developments and trends shaping the field of accreditation.

Topics regularly covered include

- how to crosswalk JCAHO, HCFA, and CARF standards;
- coordinating long-term care, subacute care, and special unit survey efforts; and
- making accreditation work as a business selling point.

Some free subscriber benefits include the following:

- "LTC Talk"—our Internet discussion group where readers can network with their peers; and
- Fax Express—whatever news happens that just can't wait, subscribers receive the pertinent information by fax so they'll always be the first to know.

Books

The Compliance Guide to the Medical Staff Standards: Winning Strategies for Your JCAHO Survey, Second Edition
by Richard E. Thompson, MD

The Compliance Guide to the Medical Staff Standards: Winning Strategies for Your JCAHO Survey, Second Edition simplifies your survey preparation efforts and even teaches you how to preserve those efforts after your survey. It explains and examines the JCAHO medical staff standards and offers advice on how to

- avoid common mistakes that can adversely affect JCAHO accreditation;
- complete survey preparation tasks that will help you gather information, share it, and use it to plan for improvement;
- review your hospital's current preparation activities for the medical staff using the provided checklists; and
- share information on the medical staff standards with medical staff leaders, the hospital's survey coordinator, and physician leaders.

Comprised of over 150 pages containing forms, checklists, and examples, this guidebook examines the 1998 medical staff standards and offers detailed advice on how to comply with them. Each chapter ranks the standards by degree of difficulty so you'll know exactly where to focus your efforts first.

How to Develop & Implement a Multidisciplinary Assessment Form

Designed to eliminate wasted time and ensure accuracy, *How to Develop & Implement a Multidisciplinary Assessment Form* provides a sample form that hospitals can use as a springboard for developing their own assessment form. Comprehensive and "patient friendly," *How to Develop & Implement a Multidisciplinary Assessment Form* will help you streamline your patient documentation efforts by creating a single form that eliminates duplication and ensures thorough and concise data collection.

The JCAHO Survey Coordinator's Handbook

Designed to walk you through the complicated survey preparation process from start to finish, *The JCAHO Survey Coordinator's Handbook* offers easy-to-understand guidelines, tips, and other valuable suggestions to help you and your organization to successfully meet JCAHO requirements. With this handbook's practical, step-by-step advice, you'll learn how to develop a survey preparation plan, review your documents and medical records for JCAHO compliance, and prepare your staff for surveyors' questions—all within your time frame.

Information Management: The Compliance Guide to the JCAHO Standards, Second Edition

This hands-on compliance guide brings the latest and most accurate health information for a JCAHO survey. It offers you a straightforward analysis of JCAHO's IM standards and includes detailed, practical advice on how to develop an information management plan, improve your medical records, and prepare your facility for JCAHO survey interviews. *Information Management* also allows you to earn 6 CE credits simply by taking the quiz in the book—at a fraction of what you would normally pay.

Leadership: The Compliance Guide to the JCAHO Standards
by Richard Schmidt Jr., JD, LLM, and Mary Becker, RRA, MBA
This book provides you with detailed interpretations and advice on how to comply with each leadership standard and other related standards. You'll learn to address the different leadership groups—the board of directors, the medical staff, the administrative team, and hospital management—and direct them in their leadership roles as defined by the JCAHO's standards.

Patient and Family Education: The Compliance Guide to the JCAHO Standards
by Joan Iacono, RN, MSN, MBA, and Ann Campbell, RN, MSN
Patient and Family Education: examines the current patient and family education (PF) and related standards for hospitals and explains them in simple, practical terms. You will learn how to develop a patient and family education program that meets the needs of your organization and its patients, and how to avoid Type I recommendations on these standards.

Performance Improvement: Winning Strategies for Quality and JCAHO Compliance
by Cynthia Barnard, MM, CPHQ, and Jodi Eisenberg, CMSC
Written by two health care quality and accreditation specialists whose hospital scored in the top 1% of hospitals nationally in a recent JCAHO survey, this book offers you a step-by-step approach to developing a strong PI program in your organization.

This book will help you to

- prioritize your PI initiatives and ensure that you focus on issues that really matter;
- determine what you do and don't need to include in your PI plan and PI program;
- demystify performance measurement and assessment;
- conduct the required PI program self-assessment once all of your improvements have en made;
  understand the new ORYX initiative;
- understand what hospital leaders' PI responsibilities are and how to garner leadership's support of your PI program;
- prepare staff and leaders for the surveyors' PI questions;
- ensure that the hospital meets Joint Commission standards; and
- prepare for the key PI-related sessions of your JCAHO survey.

Ready, Set, JCAHO! Questions, Games, and Other Strategies to Prepare Your Staff for Survey
by Candace J. Hamner, RN, MA
Ready, Set, JCAHO! was created to make your job easier. This book provides universal techniques for helping everyone be prepared and more at ease when survey day arrives. It presents simple, easy, and entertaining ways to disseminate essential information to staff throughout your

organization. From quizzes and games to theme days and contests, *Ready, Set, JCAHO!* offers both traditional and non-traditional training approaches.

Restraint and Seclusion: Improving Practice and Conquering the JCAHO Standards
by Jack Zusman, MD
This book dissects and analyzes the JCAHO's standards relating to restraint and seclusion in clear, concise language. *Restraint and Seclusion* examines the pros and cons of restraint use, presents ideas for improving patient care in your organization, and discusses issues that relate specifically to seclusion. In addition, this book will enable you to

- understand when and why restraints should be used;
- reduce the risk of physical injury and minimize psychological and social harm to patients in restraint and seclusion;
- address legal risk, patient consent, and staff education; and
- create detailed policies and procedures using the samples provided.

VIDEOS

Turning JCAHO Confusion into Confidence: How Every Employee Can Answer the JCAHO's Top Survey Questions
Geared for everyone from the CEO or nurse manager to an environmental service worker or registration clerk, *Turning JCAHO Confusion into Confidence* provides universal techniques for helping everyone in the hospital be better prepared and more at ease when survey day arrives. This 15-minute video and the accompanying training materials will teach your staff how to make a positive contribution to the hospital's survey, regardless of what role they play within the organization.

SEMINARS

Effective JCAHO Survey Preparation Seminar
You'll walk away from this seminar with practical, hands-on tools, resources, and advice on how to comply with the JCAHO standards as well as prepare for a survey. Faculty members give in-depth advice on how to avoid common Type I's by providing real-life examples that work.

Effective JCAHO Survey Preparation for the Medical Staff Seminar
With this seminar, medical staff and hospital leaders learn the critical survey issues that the entire medical staff faces. Physician leaders and key administrators also get practical ideas on the kind of medical staff involvement that will help ensure a successful survey. You will also take home clear examples of how to comply with JCAHO standards without wasting valuable time.

Consulting Services

Accreditation and Survey Preparation Consulting Services
TGC's staff has years of experience dealing with JCAHO, NCQA, and other surveys and will share our hands-on strategies. TGC consultants agree that no one approach can fit every situation—determining your specific needs is the only way to identify the most effective solutions. And because TGC is completely independent from all accrediting organizations, they interpret the standards in easy-to-understand terms.

To obtain additional information, to order any of the above products, or to comment on *The JCAHO Mock Survey Made Simple, 1999 Edition*, please contact us at:

Opus Communications
P.O. Box 1168
Marblehead, MA 01945
Toll-free telephone: 800/650-6787
Toll-free fax: 800/639-8511
E-mail: customer_service@opuscomm.com
Internet: www.opuscomm.com